Sarcoidosis - Diagnosis, Research, and Therapy of a Granulomatous Disease

Edited by Jelena Stojšić

Published in London, United Kingdom

Sarcoidosis - Diagnosis, Research, and Therapy of a Granulomatous Disease
http://dx.doi.org/10.5772/intechopen.1000413
Edited by Jelena Stojšić

Contributors
Deepak Rosha, Inês S.F. da Silva, Ryan Costa Silva, Inês Sopa, Lígia Peixoto, Lily Lebwohl, Robert G. Phelps, Abhishek Sethi, Corrina P. Azarcon, Monique Munro, Francesco Rastelli, Luisa Benozzi, Stefano Cusinato, Marilena Stoian, Cedric Pluguez-Turull, Cinthia Del Toro, Youley Tjendra, Alicia K. Gerke

First published in London, United Kingdom, 2024 by IntechOpen
IntechOpen is the global imprint of INTECHOPEN LIMITED, registered in England and Wales, registration number: 11086078, 5 Princes Gate Court, London, SW7 2QJ, United Kingdom

British Library Cataloguing-in-Publication Data
A catalogue record for this book is available from the British Library

Additional hard and PDF copies can be obtained from orders@intechopen.com

Sarcoidosis - Diagnosis, Research, and Therapy of a Granulomatous Disease
Edited by Jelena Stojšić
p. cm.
Print ISBN 978-1-83769-953-7
Online ISBN 978-1-83769-952-0
eBook (PDF) ISBN 978-1-83769-954-4

Meet the editor

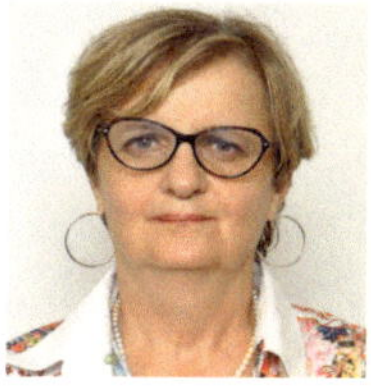

Jelena Stojšić is a senior scientific researcher and has been a thoracic pathologist for the last 28 years. His major interests include lung pathology, lung cancer, and interstitial lung diseases, especially sarcoidosis. She has researched genetic alterations in lung cancer and their impact on personalized therapy. She has given many invited speeches and is the author of many articles on sarcoidosis. She is also an editor of journal special issues and books.

Contents

Preface

This book is dedicated to modern understandings of sarcoidosis as well as already-known aspects of the disease. It presents new, modern information on the etiology of sarcoidosis and its clinical manifestations depending on the affected organs. The diagnosis of sarcoidosis is a unique challenge and requires clinical-pathological and radiological correlation, which is discussed throughout some chapters. The book also discusses therapy for this disease.

This book is intended for general practitioners, internists, pulmonologists, and other medical specialists, such as dentists, ophthalmologists, and dermatologists.

Jelena Stojšić, MD Ph.D.
University Clinical Centre of Serbia,
Belgrade, Serbia

Chapter 1

A Hypothesis to Explain the Genesis of Sarcoidosis

Deepak Rosha

Abstract

Sarcoidosis is a disease of immune cell dysfunction. This review serves to amalgamate the information available into a coherent hypothesis. Recent research has shown that sarcoidosis should not be considered an antigenic induced granulomatous disease alone. The contribution of activation of auto immunity also has to be recognised. The triggering antigens have been narrowed mostly to be derived from *Mycobacterial* tubercular proteins and *Propionobacter acnes*. It is possible that they may share a common particle that creates a conformational change in the receptors of Th-1 cells that drives the disease until there is switch to autoimmunity and subsequent development of fibrosis. The role of genetic and environmental factors is also reviewed in this context.

Keywords: sarcoidosis, genesis, hypothesis, granulomagens, autoimmunity

1. Introduction

Sarcoidosis has remained an enigmatic disease since its description by Hutchinson, and subsequent reporting of histopathology by Boeck more than a 100 years ago [1]. Extensive research from many countries has produced voluminous information.

We know that sarcoidosis is an immune disorder where epithelioid non-caseating granulomas form early in the disease with later development of fibrosis if the disease persists. There is a predilection for the lungs and mediastinal lymph-nodes but the disorder can involve any organ of the body. We also know that it involves Th1/Th2/Th17 type responses from the CD4+ T-helper cells, which are typically provoked by difficult to degrade antigens. In addition there is dysregulation of suppressor responses [2]. The problem is that no antigen has been consistently found in the sarcoid tissue, although remnant proteins of the *Mycobacterium* species have been identified in approximately 20–60% of the tissues tested in various studies. Another putative organism is *Propionobacter acnes* which has also been detected in upto 85% sarcoid tissue. This is also the only organism to have been cultured from sarcoid granulomas [3]. Although many studies have detected this bacteria, others have not, leaving its causative nature in doubt. Many other antigens like fungi, pollens and other organic material have been considered and discarded for the present. A similar disease can be produced on exposure Beryllium, Zirconium, Silica and other inorganic particles [4].

The Kviem test had shown that a transmissible agent or factor is present in the sarcoid tissue, as this can produce granulomas when injected into the subcutaneous tissues of another sarcoid patient. To be noted is that non-sarcoid tissue when injected into the same patient would not produce a similar response [5]. A tuberculin test at 6 weeks may also produce a similar response in a sarcoid patient, but not other injected proteins. The transmissible granulomagenic factor(GF) can be destroyed by heating the sarcoid tissue at high temperature, but not by heating at lower temperatures [6].

It has also been noted that sarcoidosis may develop in donor lung transplant, if the recipient has sarcoidosis [7]. Sarcoidosis has been reported to occur in recipient of stem cell transplant if the donor had sarcoidosis. Donor immune cells have been identified in the granuloma in this situation [8].

Cases of sarcoidosis have been seen more frequently clustered in families, leading to the consideration that genetic and environmental factors are important. The severity of sarcoidosis and organs involved vary in different regions and ethnic groups. These features have been linked to genetic variations especially HLA class II alleles although other genetic loci are also implicated [9].

In areas of high *Mycobacterium* tuberculosis transmission, it has been reported that some patients of tuberculosis go on to develop sarcoidosis, the reverse has also been reported. This entity has been termed 'Tuberculo-sarcoid'. Thus there is evidence that some form of altered *Mycobacterial* protein is a contender for the initiation and genesis of sarcoidosis [10]. It has been reported in bronchoalveolar lavage fluid (BALF) of sarcoidosis patients that T lymphocytes are very reactive to mycobacterial peptides namely 6-kDa, early secreted antigenic protein (ESAT-6) or catalase peroxide (KatG) [11].

The heavy metal Beryllium and other inorganic substances like silica and Zircon can produce a sarcoid like granulomatous disorder. But these are distinct from sarcoidosis as they can be distinguished by laboratory tests [12].

The fact that anti- inflammatory treatment by Gluco-corticoids or cytotoxic drugs like Methotrexate and not antibiotic or anti tubercular treatment cause improvement and even remission in the disease, highlights that the disease is not caused by an actively multiplying intact organism [13].

2. Granuloma formation in sarcoidosis

Granuloma formation is a specific body response where the immune system has to deal with difficult to degrade or non-biodegradable granulomagenic factor (GF). The granulomagen is first taken up as part of an antigen by the receptors of an antigen presenting cell (APC). These are dendritic cells and macrophages. This foreign substance is recognised as non self, and presented by Th-1 cells that display genetically determined HLA class II antigens to macrophages that ingest the particle and try to destroy it by enzymatic action. Being unable to carry out this task they secrete various factors and interleukins that signal between cells calling upon more cells to enter the involved field. Areas that appear like a ball of nucleated cells develop. Some of the macrophages coalesce to form giant cells and accumulate to form the typical granulomatous tissue. The conglomerate of epithelioid and multinucleate giant cells in the center, surrounded by lymphocytes of the CD4+ type and rare CD8+ T cells as well as some B cells in the periphery has given rise to the terminology epithelioid granulomas. In the case of some granulomas there may be associated vascular involvement and tissue necrosis. In other cases as in *M. TUB.* there may be caseous destruction of the tissue. The sarcoid granulomas are well formed with distinctive giant cells and necrosis is usually absent [14].

3. Initiation of sarcoid granulomas

There is a distinct polymorphism within genes that code for proteins involved in T cell activation, differentiation, proliferation and persistence which include ANXA11 and NOTCH 4. Risk factors have also been associated within the antigen presentation gene locus 6p21.3 that encode for proteins involved in T cell regulation and antigen presentation involving both HLA and butyrophilin like protein BTNL 2 receptors [15].

On the first exposure to antigen there is the development of tissue hypersensitivity which may or may not be clinically obvious. The macrophages and antigen presenting cells (APC) which are constituted mainly by dendritic cells (DC) are primed. Further exposure to the antigen causes the DC to pick up the antigens and migrate to the local lymph nodes (LN). Here the DC initiate specific T cell differentiation and proliferation. The macrophages also contribute to the early recognition of the antigen in the lung and secrete chemokines such as RANTES, MIP-1 alpha and beta. The Macrophages in addition produce pro inflammatory cytokines such as Interleukin-1 (IL-1) and TNF-alpha, The monocytes highly express Toll like receptor (TLR-2) and also produce TNF-alpha, IL-1beta, and IL-6 when stimulated by ligands ESAT-6, KatG, and endogenous Amyloid A. These activities produce a further influx of monocytes, and LN activated lymphocytes leading to CD4+ alveolitis if the portal of entry is into the lung [16].

The APC with the antigen in the receptor site induce persisting stimulation of the immune cells mediated by HLA related proteins leading to continuous expansion of macrophages and lymphocytes and ultimately to granuloma formation.

4. Persistence of granuloma

The role of TNF-alpha is very important in granuloma formation and persistence. The TNF-alpha produces macrophage activation, migration and leucocyte adhesion. The alveolar macrophages when stimulated by TNF-alpha, and IL-1beta produce CCL20 which is a chemokine attracting DC's, B cells and specific T-cells towards the site of inflammation. TNF-alpha is also needed for leucocyte adhesion giving rise to high density of cells. This adhesion is induced by intercellular adhesion molecule (ICAM-1).

Following adhesion the histiocyte epithelioid cells and monocyte derived DC's can fuse to form multinucleated giant cells in the presence of TNF-alpha, GM CSF, IL-17A, CCL20 and interferon -gamma. This process is assisted by natural killer cells that produce INF-gamma.

Differentiation of the T cells is dependent on the cytokines associated with the APCs. Th1 and Th17 differentiation is driven in the presence of INF-alpha, IL-2, IL-17. Further Th1 differentiation also depends on IL-12 and IL-18 whereas Th17 is driven by IL-6 and TGF-beta, but the survival and proliferation of Th17 is also dependent on IL-23. It should be noted that IL-17A/IFN-gamma and IL-17A/IL-4 producing cells are seen to be increased in the peripheral blood of active sarcoidosis. Such a picture is also found in auto immune disease. B cells and plasma cells are present surrounding the granuloma and there are increased serum levels of B cell activating factor (BAFF). These features may select auto reactive B cells leading to antibody production. ANA positivity may be seen in 30–60% of sarcoidosis patients.

There is additional dysfunction of the T regulator cell(T-regs). In Sarcoidosis the T-regs fail to inhibit TNF-alpha, INF-gamma, and IL-2 that contribute to granuloma formation. This ability is restored on recovery.

Recovery from the granulomatous disease may take place with or without tissue destruction depending on the granulomagen. Tuberculosis may heal with fibrosis and distortion of local tissue. On the other-hand sarcoidosis may heal spontaneously or have remission and exacerbations or they may be progressive fibrosis. The destruction of tissue in tuberculosis is due to tissue hypersensitivity but in sarcoidosis the persistent granulomas ultimately cause the invasion of fibroblasts and fibrosis [17].

Anti inflammatory treatment in sarcoidosis elicits a variable response that is dependent on host, environmental factors and possibly the extent of immune dysregulation.

The mode of entry of the granulomagen is commonly into the lung parenchyma from where it may or may not spread via lymphatics to other parts of the body, the other commonly involved organ is the skin [18].

5. The Kviem test

Although the Kviem test is no longer in use now, it has generated much speculation for its enigmatic features. Essentially the test entails harvesting sarcoid material from the spleen of a patient. The tissue is then purified by exposure to various chemicals and heating as well as centrifugation and irradiation. Subsequently it is injected into a suspected case of sarcoidosis. A test is considered positive if a papule develops over 6 weeks, which on biopsy shows non-caseating granulomas.

The test is positive however in about 60% cases in early sarcoidosis and in those after 2 years of disease, true positivity declines to about 20–30%. The waning of this response has not been adequately explained.

The Kviem particle which may be causing the granulomatous response has not been detected despite intense investigation including the use of polymerase chain reaction (PCR} and immunohistochemistry (IHC). However what is known is that Kviem reactivity is nullified if the harvested tissue is exposed to strong acids, alkali, high heat and even centrifugation at high RPM.

The Kviem particle does not appear to lose potency even if tissue from the same papule is injected a few more times into the same subject. Suggesting the persistence of a GF.

At the time when intense immune activity is taking place in the sarcoid patient a seemingly paradoxical cutaneous anergy develops. This can be explained by dysregulated suppressor activity on the appropriate reacting cells.

As the disease progresses, the Kviem test becomes negative probably as the there is a switch in host to activity of the immune system towards autoimmunity against autoantigens and producing fibrosis. At this point the GF polarised T cells diminish as does granuloma formation [19].

6. Genetics in sarcoidosis

The role of genetics in sarcoidosis has been extensively studied in various ethnic groups. The role of class I HLA alleles as well as Class II DR alleles, and non HLA genes have been investigated. From our own studies in Indian patients and their comparison with other ethnic groups we can say that within ethnic groups certain genes either appear to be protective or increase the risk but the same cannot necessarily be extended to other groups. Probably there are genes in linkage disequilibrium that are confounding the issue [20]. The role of genetics is further discussed under Lofgrens syndrome.

7. Non infectious risk factors

Several studies have linked sarcoidosis to the exposure of non infectious agents. It is possible that these agents may act either as adjuvants that trigger the disease in a predisposed individual or are directly causative. Sarcoidosis is more commonly seen in spring from which one could point to pollens or other abundant bio-aerosols that may occur at that time. Of note is a sarcoid like disease seen in fire fighters exposed to combustible substances. Additionally there have been reports of association between toner in printer ink and sarcoidosis. Some of those exposed to the dust from collapse of the world trade center also developed sarcoidosis in a significantly large number, but it is not clear if the inciting agent was dust metal particles or gas. The Sarcoid like disease caused by Beryllium and other inert inorganic substances has already been mentioned [21].

Intuitively inert substances may act as adjuvants rather than actual inciting antigens, because a repeated and adequately heavy exposure would be required for the disease to be initiated and maintained. We already have mentioned that *P acnes* may multiply in macrophages to increase the antigenic load. Similarly a latent *M tub*. infection may become active and then after an initial phase of multiplication, the bacteria may degenerate for unknown reasons, leaving enough antigen to incite a granulomatosis response [22].

8. Auto immunity and sarcoidosis

The hall mark of sarcoidosis is the non caseating granuloma and the well described Th1 response. In the core of the granuloma are macrophages, giant cells, CD3+/CD4+ T -helper cells, whereas in the outer portion CD+8 T lymphocytes, T-Regs, fibroblasts and B-lymphocytes predominate. The T-helper type 1 produce gamma-interferon that is essential to induce and maintain macrophage activation leading to chronic disease.

The recent discovery of T-helper 17 cells and its highly specialised sub type Th1/Th17 capable of producing Interleukin 17 and Gamma Interferon both in the local sites and peripheral blood thus reducing the T-regs in the granulomas and increasing them in the systemic circulation has improved the understanding of the immune dysregulation. The 17 cells also contribute to fibrosis and may reflect a switch from external antigen stimulation to auto antigens notably Vimentin [23].

Another notable feature is that Macrophages begin to differentiate to M-2 type which contribute to chronicity by their pro fibrotic and anti inflammatory properties [24].

It seems reasonable to propose that progressive sarcoidosis is characterised by continuous immune dysregulation long after the triggering antigens cannot be detected. This could happen if

a. a granulomagenic factor derived from the triggering antigen persist in the receptor pockets of the Th-1 causing a conformational change that drives the response

b. over time the driving T-helper cells become autonomous due to their genotype even as the GF disappears.

c. there is exposure to self antigens as tissue damage progresses with the development of a switch to auto immunity that drives the disease to fibrosis.

9. The Lofgrens and Heerfordt's syndrome

The Lofgrens syndrome characterised by fever, arthralgia, arthritis, uveitis, erythema nodosum and bilateral hilar lymphadenopathy is considered to be an early form of sarcoidosis. Many of these cases resolve but a substantial number go on to develop sarcoidosis. A similar syndrome may be seen in tuberculosis called Poncet's disease [25]. Erythema nodosum can also been seen in leprosy, streptococcal disease, rickettsial disease and exposure to some other infectious organisms. Biopsy of the erythema nodosum shows a septal panniculitis common to all with infiltration with macrophages and lymphocytes. There is no granuloma formation, and no organisms seen. Thus these constellation of signs and symptoms should be considered to be the priming of the immune system, with development of tissue hypersensitivity [26]. A similar reaction in Heerfodt's syndrome causing parotid enlargement and facial paralysis can be also similarly considered, only the portal of entry being different. A significant point to note here is that many patients may be asymptomatic.

The commonest portals of entry are Lungs and skin of the inciting antigens that contain the GF. Once the first experience of the naive immune system is established, the primed immune cells spread via lymphatics to sites that are pre- determined. These sites are not unique to LS and exhibit similar response to other antigens in which DTH develops. A non specific inflammation is set up. This inflammation may subside over time with treatment or spontaneously. This is attributed to an appropriately functioning immune suppressor system [27].

It is seen that the Class II alleles HLA-DRB-1*03 and DQB1*0201 located in the antigen presenting cells are commonly associated with LS and their presence is prognostically favourable for the reaction to subside. These alleles are seen in patients with LS in Scandinavia. On the other hand in Japan the presence of HLA-DRB1*04 is often associated with Uveitis [28].

In our study in Asian Indians we found these alleles to be rare and LS as well as sarcoidosis associated Uveitis to be uncommon. However we often see Uveitis associated with strongly positive tuberculin test that responds well to anti-tubercular treatment. The genetics of this latter manifestation however have not been adequately studied [29].

Alternatively due to dysregulation of suppressor cells, the disease may progress to the next stage which is of granuloma formation. Associated alleles of the class II genes HLA-DRB1*15, HLA-DRB1*07, HLA-DRB1*14 are often present in the genotype in the APC's that lead to progressive and chronic sarcoidosis. However in African- Americans who are predisposed to a severe type of sarcoidosis the allele HLA- DRB1*1101 is commonly seen. These alleles express their proteins in the pockets that form in the T helper cells and contain receptors to foreign antigens. In our study we found that HLA- DRB1*15 to be associated with a good prognosis in Asian Indians. But as in other studies, HLA-DRB1*14 and HLA-DRB1*07 were linked to progressive disease [30].

10. Discussion

A number of derivations from the above information can be now presented

1. All antigens that produce Sarcoidosis contain a granulomagenic factor (GF), that persists in sarcoid tissue even if the antigen itself disintegrates. The GF remains intact over long periods of time if it remains in the cell wall but may be disintegrate once in the interstitium.

2. The granulomagenic factor incorporates itself in the pocket of the receptor located in the membrane of the Th1 cells and macrophages. This produces dysregulation and autonomy of the Th1 /Th17 cells. These cells then spread to various organs, where they attract macrophages and cause the macrophages to produce cell signalling interleukins, cytokines and other factors that attract more macrophages to ultimately develop the granuloma.

3. If the sarcoid tissue is now injected into another sarcoid patient the granulomagenic factor is released from dying macrophages and T-helper cells. The GF retains the capacity to promote further formation of local granulomas (for some time} and is incorporated into the host receptors of Th cells.

4. This also explains the granulomagenecity of the tuberculin test. But the occurrence of sarcoidosis in donor lung in a transplanted recipient patient of sarcoidosis is due to the dissemination of the autonomous and dysregulated host Th cells into the tissue.

5. The persistence of disease depends on a number of factors including genetic and environmental factors. After the initial exposure to the antigen, a tissue hypersensitivity develops. The antigen load will determine the GF load. The organism may initially multiply within the host tissues and later degenerate releasing the antigen. The interaction between the GF and the macrophages and Th cells will now determine the dissemination of the cells to other tissues and their progressive dysregulation where suppressor cells become unable to dampen the spread and granuloma formation [31].

6. The GF is probably a nano or submicroscopic particle in the macrophages and in the altered pocket of the T cell receptors [32]. The GF is probably common in structure despite being derived from differing inciting antigens.

7. The further course will depend on the load of the GF in tissues, apoptosis of the cells may cause the disease to regress if GF load is low. But if the GF load is high apoptosis may be prevented by the presence of the GF and granulomas then persist.

8. As mentioned above the T helper cells also become autonomous aided by a dysregulation of suppressor cells, and continue to initiate granuloma formation. Even after the initiating GF has disintegrated, M-2 macrophages may target auto antigens leading to regression of granulomas and development of progressive fibrosis.

9. Anti inflammatory drugs like glucocorticoids may cause lymphocyte apoptosis leading to extrusion of the GF from macrophages and other granuloma forming cells into the interstitium where it may persist for some time. Glucocorticoids also inhibit the uptake of the GF by macrophages. For this reason there may be a relapse if the glucocorticoids are given for too short a time. Glucocorticoids may also restore the function of the suppressor cells, allowing a restoration of the balance between the effector and suppressor cells.
   Thus the inability of the body to switch off the granuloma response, may be reversed by anti- inflammatory action of glucocorticoids.

10. If the disease progresses unchecked there is now a switch to increased M2 macrophage activity that targets autoantigens and promotes fibrosis. At this point the host loses the Kviem reactivity, as the disease becomes more autoimmune and Th cell activity driven by GF declines. In this regard self antigens have been identified to which the immune system becomes reactive, most notably Vimentin. The protein Amyloid A also plays a role.

11. The reason why the genesis of sarcoidosis has been difficult to understand is because of the changes that take place over time. To put it all together

    a. there is the initial phase of hypersensitivity as seen in Lofgrens syndrome, a similar Poncets disease is seen in Tuberculosis. This signifies an initial exposure to the antigen and priming of the immune system.

    b. At this stage many factors begin to play a role. The major components are genetic most notably the Class II DR alleles. Another factor may be the antigen load. There may be a requirement for high level of antigen exposure for the disease to be progressive. *P acnes* has been seen to proliferate inside macrophages without causing overt disease but at the same time inducing a spread of bacteria and a strong cellular response. *Mycobacteria* may do the same but both degenerate for unknown reasons leaving their antigens behind.

    c. If the suppressor cells are effective and the antigen exposure below a threshold the disease will subside when in the early stages.

    d. For the disease to progress, adequate amount GF gets incorporated into the receptors of T-helper CD-4 cells, this promotes the granuloma forming cascade. This also causes a proliferation of the Th-1/Th-17 phenotype. At this point the Kviem test would be positive if this tissue is injected into another sarcoid patient because the GF factor can be taken up by the host cells.

    e. Again over a period of time the concerned T cells develop a permanent conformational change that cause two effects: one an unsuppressed proliferation of the polarised Th cells and second: dissemination of these cells to other organs. *Notably by this time the original GF has disintegrated and is no longer needed for the disease to continue.*

    f. Persistence of the disease now promotes fibrosis. There is once again a change in the immune state this time from granulomatous to an autoimmune pathogenesis. The macrophages shift to the M2 type and the Th2 responses begin to predominate with the production of auto antibodies.

    g. Thus the reason for the difficulty in understanding sarcoidosis has been to classify it in a single slot i.e. a granulomatous disease, where as it should be seen as progressing through tissue hypersensitivity to granuloma initiated by antigen but maintained by a granulomagenic factor, followed by autonomous T helper cells proliferation causing dissemination of granuloma forming cells to other organs and finally a switch to auto-immune disease leading to tissue fibrosis

h. The granulomagenic particle cannot be detected by immunohistochemistry or PCR because it is a nano particle derived from the antigens to which the host was initially exposed.

11. The hypothesis

The granulomagen probably has a common structural configuration that is found in several antigens including the *Mycobacterial* cell wall. This GF which is also transmissible probably incorporates itself into the membrane receptors of the Th-1 cells and inside macrophages causing the secretion of cytokine, chemoattractants and interleukins and increasing the local cellularity of immune cells.

Being deeply embedded into the T cell receptors and thus incorporated as a part of the membrane, the GF is no longer extractable or identifiable even by polymerase chain reaction or immunohistochemistry. We postulate that the macrophages of the sarcoidosis patient that are circulating are primed or sensitised to the granulomagen even though not participating in the granuloma formation. There is also inappropriate suppressor cell activity that causes a loss of skin hypersensitivity to common antigens.

The GF, when injected into the tissue of a sarcoid patient, although present in the membrane of donor Th-1 and inside macrophages may be released by destruction of these very macrophages in the host tissue, after which they get incorporated into the host macrophages that are already primed. In this way granulomas begin to be locally produced by exciting the release of interleukins and signalling factors.

We have deliberately avoided the term 'Antigen' and replaced it by 'Granulomagen', which we postulate is a submicroscopic particle common to all antigens that have the capability to produce granulomas. In Berylliosis the Kviem test was found to be negative so we can say with confidence that even though the granuloma produced by Berylliosis is similar, it is not the same.

The tuberculin test may also produce granulomas at the injection site, at 6 weeks in a patient of sarcoidosis. This points to the granulomagen present in the tuberculin protein.

12. Conclusion

Sarcoidosis should be considered to be a disease of immune cell dysfunction, provoked in a susceptible individual by an antigen that is a part of a microbe capable of multiplication and subsequent degeneration. The granulomagenic factor contained in this antigen is translocated into the receptors of CD4+ Th1 cells where it generates the granulomatous response. Overtime the Th1 cells of this polarity become autonomous, escaping the immune suppression by T regulatory cells. In the final phase the Th1/Th17 cellular response dominates where the disease switches to self antigens and becomes autoimmune leading to fibrosis.

Author details

Deepak Rosha
Institute of Respiratory, Critical Care and Sleep Medicine, Indraprastha Apollo Hospitals, New Delhi, India

*Address all correspondence to: deepakrosha@gmail.com

References

[1] Spagnolo P. Sarcoidosis: A critical review of history and milestones. Clinical Reviews in Allergy and Immunology. 2015;**49**:1-5

[2] Beijer E, Veltcamp M, Meek B. Etiology and immunopathogenesis of sarcoidosis: Novel insights. Seminars in Respiratory and Critical Care Medicine. 2017;**38**(04):404-416

[3] Yamaguchi T, Costabel U, McDowell A, et al. Immunohistochemical detection of potential microbial antigens in granulomas in the diagnosis of sarcoidosis. Journal of Clinical Medicine. 2021;**10**:983

[4] Judson MA. Environmental risk factors for sarcoidosis. Frontier in Immunology. 2020;**11**:1340

[5] Munro CS, Mitchell DN, Poulter LW, et al. Early cellular responses to intradermal injection of Kveim suspensions in normal subjects and those with sarcoidosis. Journal of Clinical Pathology. 1986;**39**:176-182

[6] Jayashree P, Ashique KT, Nair NG. Tuberculin skin test reaction and sarcoidosis - an unexpected sequela. Indian Dermatology Online Journal. 2020;**11**(3):431-432

[7] Padila ML, Schilero GJ, Teirstein AS. Donor acquired sarcoidosis. Sarcoidosis, Vasculitis and Diffuse Lung Disease. 2002;**19**(1):18-24

[8] Kushima H, Ishii H, Ikewaki J, et al. Sarcoidosis in donor derived tissues after haematopetic stem cell transplantation. European Respiratory Journal. 2013;**41**(6):1452-1453

[9] Rossman MD, Thompson B, Fredrick M, et al. HLA and enviofrnmental interactionin sarcoidosis. Sarcoidosis, Vasculitis, and Diffuse Lung Diseases. 2008;**25**:125-132

[10] Shah JR, Hede J, Mathur RS. Diagnostic criteria of tuberculous-sarcoidosis. Lung India. 2009;**26**:86-88

[11] Oswald-Richter KA, Culver D, Hawkins C, et al. Cellular responses to mycobacterial antigens are present in broncheoalveolar lavage fluid used in the diagnosis of sarcoidosis. Infection and Immunology. 2009;**77**(9):3740-3748

[12] Newman LS, Rose CS, Bresnitz EA, et al. A case control etiological study of sarcoidosis: Environmental and occupational risk factors. American Journal of Respiratory Critical Care Medicine. 2004;**170**:1324-1330

[13] Planey SL, Litwack G. Glucocorticoid induced apoptosis in lymphocytes. Biochemical and Biophysical Research Communications. 2000;**279**(2):307-312

[14] Broos CE, van Nimwegen C, Hoogsteden HC, et al. Granuloma formation in pulmonary sarcoidosis. Frontiers in Immunology. 2013;**4**:437

[15] Rybicki BA, Waleski JL, Maliarik MJ, et al. The BTNL2 gene and sarcoid susceptibility in African Americans and Whites. American Journal of Human Genetics. 2005;**77**(3):491-499

[16] Rosen Y, Athanassiades TJ, Moon S, et al. Non granulomatous interstitial pneumonitis in sarcoidosis. Relationship to development of epithelioid granulomas. Chest. 1978;**74**(2):122-125

[17] Wilson JL, Hk M, Weichart T. Metabolic programming of macrophages implications in the pathogenesis of

granulomatous disease. Frontier in Immunology. 2019;**10**:2265

[18] Baughman RP, Tierstein AS, Judson MA, et al. Clinical characteristics of patients in a case control study of sarcoidosis. American Journal of Respiratory Critical Care Medicine. 2001;**164**(10):1885-1889

[19] Munro CS, Mithchell DN. The Kveim response: Still useful still a puzzle. Thorax. 1987;**42**:321-331

[20] Rosha D, Chowdhry M, Gupta I. Influence of HLA class II DRBI*/DQBI* allles in phenotypes of Indian patients of sarcoidosis. European Respiratory Journal. 2021;**58**:703

[21] Barnard J, Rose C, Newman L, et al. Job and industry classifications associated with sarcoidosis in a case control etiological study of sarcoidosis (ACCESS). Journal of Occupational Environmental Medicine. 2005;**47**:226-234

[22] Hernandez-Pando R, Jeyanathan M, Mengistu G, et al. Persistence of DNA from *Mycobacterium tuberculosis* in superficially normal lung tissue during latent infection. Lancet. 2000;**356**:2133-2138

[23] Starshinva AA, Malkova AM, Basantova NY, et al. Sarcoidosis as an autoimmune disease. Frontier in Immunology. 2020;**10**:2933

[24] Shamaei M, Mortaz E, Pourabdollah M, et al. Evidence for M2 macrophages in granulomas from pulmonary sarcoidosis: A new aspect of macrophage heterogenicity. Human Immunology. 2018;**79**:63-69

[25] Dall L, Long L, Stanford J. Poncets disease: Tuberculous rheumatism. Review in Infectious Diseases. 1989;**11**:105-107

[26] Perez-Garza DM, Chavez-Alvarez S, Ocampio-Candiani J, et al. Erythema Nodosum: A practical approach and diagnostic algorithm. American Journal of Clinical Dermatology. 2021;**22**(3):367-378

[27] Zissel G, Prasse A, Mueller-Quernheim J. Immunological response of sarcoidosis. Seminars in Respiratory Critical Care Medicine. 2010;**31**(4):390-403

[28] Grunewald J. Review: Role of genetics in susceptibility and outcomes of sarcoidosis. Seminars in Respiratory Critical Care Medicine. 2010;**31**(4):380-389

[29] Agarwal R, Gunasekran DV, Grany R, et al. Clinical features and outcomes of patients with tubercular uveitis treated with anti tubercular treatment in the collaborative ocular study (cots)1. JAMA Opthalmology. 2017;**135**(12):1318-1327

[30] Bogunia-Kubik K, Tomecsko J, Suchniki L, et al. HLA DRB1*03 Drb1*11 or DRB1*12 and their respective DrB3 specificities in clinical varieties of sarcoidosis. Tissue Antigens. 2001;**57**:87-90

[31] Grunewald J, Eklund A. Role of CD4 T cells in sarcoidosis. American Thoracic Society. 2007;**4**:461-464

[32] Hefner DK. The cause of sarcoidosis: The centurial enigma solved. Annals of Diagnostic Pathology. 2007;**11**(2):142-152

Chapter 2

Clinical Manifestations of Sarcoidosis

Inês S.F. da Silva, Ryan Costa Silva, Inês Sopa and Lígia Peixoto

Abstract

Sarcoidosis is a granulomatous disease characterized by granulomatous inflammation in affected tissues. Any tissue may become affected and so different symptoms can occur. There can also be asymptomatic organ involvement. It may present as a multisystem disease or individual organ involvement and it is also associated with general symptoms like fever, weight loss, night sweats or fatigue. Clinical onset may be acute or subacute and clinical course may be self-remitting or chronic. Most commonly sarcoidosis affects the lungs (manifesting as dyspnea, chest pain or cough) and/or thoracic lymph nodes. Extrapulmonary sarcoidosis includes peripheral lymphadenopathy, abdominal (including renal, hepatic, splenic, gastrointestinal), neurological, musculoskeletal, ocular, cardiac, cutaneous and head and neck sarcoidosis (including nose/paranasal sinuses, salivary glands). Less commonly, sarcoidosis can affect bone marrow. Multiple associations of organ involvement occur to configure clinical phenotypes (based on organ manifestations that frequently occur together) and syndromes like Löfgren's or Heerfordt-Waldenström's.

Keywords: clinical symptoms, pulmonary sarcoidosis, lymphadenopathy, abdominal sarcoidosis, neurosarcoidosis, skin changes

1. Introduction

Sarcoidosis is a granulomatous disease of so far unknown etiology [1] that is characterized by the development of noncaseating [2] granulomatous inflammation in affected tissues [3]. Any tissue may become affected [3] and so different symptoms/signs can occur leading to a wide range of clinical manifestations. It may present as multisystem disease or individual organ involvement and there can also be asymptomatic organ involvement.

Sarcoidosis cohorts are not homogeneous, and differ in terms of age, sex, ethnicity, type of onset and organ involvement. Clinical onset may be acute or subacute, acute onset is nevertheless rare [3]. There are more female patients affected by sarcoidosis (3:2 female/male ratio) but in patients aged ≤40 years or with subacute onset, the ratio is almost 1:1. Sarcoidosis is not only a disease of young adults, it is also frequently diagnosed in middle-aged and elderly patients. However, there are more females diagnosed during the fifth decade while males are diagnosed earlier, between the third and fourth decades [1].

 IntechOpen

The clinical course of sarcoidosis ranges from spontaneous resolution to disabling chronic disease, with lung transplantation as the last resort [1]. Around 30% of cases resolve within 2 years, particularly with single system involvement, 30% have a relapsing form and 30% progressively deteriorate. Over time, the mortality rate is greater than in the general population, relating predominantly to the severity of the disease in those with respiratory, cardiac and neurological involvement, but also to an increased risk of infection. Patients with sarcoidosis also have several other morbidities, such as venous thromboembolism, cardiovascular disease and hematological and skin cancers and a higher prevalence of other autoimmune diseases, in particular thyroid disease, connective tissue diseases and multiple sclerosis [3]. The prognosis is worst for African Americans, those with multiorgan involvement and disease onset after the age of 40 years [4].

2. Clinical manifestations of sarcoidosis

Clinical manifestations of sarcoidosis differ according to the type of onset [1], race, sex, age [5] and organ involvement.

Regarding the type of onset, patients with acute sarcoidosis significantly report more fatigue, fever, night sweats and arthralgia, but less cough and dyspnea than patients with subacute sarcoidosis. Patients with acute sarcoidosis are younger, female and more often have bronchial and musculoskeletal involvement, a radiologically normal lung and better lung function. These patients also have less frequent cardiac, hepatic or splenic involvement [1].

The extent and frequency of organ involvement varies in different ethnicities [1]. For example, African Americans suffer more often from ocular, bone marrow, extrathoracic lymph nodes and skin involvement other than erythema nodosum (NS) [5] and the disease was also found to be more severe in these subjects [6].

Male and female patients' characteristics also differ significantly: female patients suffer less from fever but suffer more from fatigue, arthralgia, chest pain, and from eye, salivary gland and skin involvement than males.

Age is an important factor influencing the clinical phenotype of patients with sarcoidosis: younger patients present predominantly with Scadding type I, whereas higher frequencies of Scadding type III or IV are noted in older patients. Patients aged ≤40 years are more prone to fever, eye, intrathoracic lymph node and bronchial involvement, but suffer less from dyspnea and heart involvement compared with patients aged >40 years [1]. Sarcoidosis has distinct characteristics in elderly people compared with younger subjects. The female-to-male ratio is higher in elderly-onset sarcoidosis (onset of sarcoidosis in people over 65 years of age), constitutional symptoms, specific skin lesions and uveitis are more frequent and erythema nodosum or asymptomatic chest X-ray abnormalities are less common compared with younger patients [7].

Finally, regarding organ involvement, pulmonary and extrapulmonary sarcoidosis can be distinguished [1]. Within pulmonary sarcoidosis, lung affection and mediastinal/hilar lymphadenopathy can be distinguished and within the extrapulmonary group it is possible to distinguish between peripheral lymphadenopathy, abdominal sarcoidosis (including renal, hepatic, splenic, gastrointestinal), neurological, musculoskeletal, ocular, cardiac, bone marrow, cutaneous and head and neck sarcoidosis (including eyes, nose/paranasal sinuses, salivary glands). Multiple organ involvement associations even configure clinical phenotypes and syndromes.

2.1 Pulmonary sarcoidosis

Most commonly sarcoidosis affects the lungs followed by mediastinal and/or hilar lymphadenopathy [1].

2.1.1 Lung sarcoidosis

Pulmonary manifestation is by far the most common organ involvement in sarcoidosis [1]. At some point, 90% of patients have abnormal chest radiographs [8].

Lung involvement is characterized by cough, breathlessness and chest tightness or stabbing pains, but is often asymptomatic [3]. Scadding's classification defines five stages of sarcoidosis on a chest radiography [9]. The most frequent type is Scadding I (bilateral hilar lymphadenopathy (BHL)) or II (BHL and pulmonary infiltrates in upper lobes). A significant number of patients do not have sarcoidosis-associated chest radiography findings (Scadding type 0) and the less frequent Scadding types are III (pulmonary infiltrates without BHL) and IV, with the latter being the least frequent, which means that signs of lung fibrosis are the least frequent finding in patients with lung sarcoidosis [1]. Pulmonary nodules tend to be termed "micronodules," ranging from 2 to 5 mm, typically located along the bronchovascular bundles, interlobular septa, interlobar fissures and subpleural regions [9]. Pulmonary function is only marginally impaired, with forced expiratory volume in 1 second (FEV1) [1] and forced vital capacity (FVC) [9] being the most reduced measures. The more advanced the radiological stage, the greater the decline in functional status [2]. Pulmonary arterial hypertension can be a serious complication in sarcoidosis [9] and occurs in 1 to 6% of patients [8].

2.1.2 Thoracic lymph nodes

Bilateral hilar lymphadenopathy is the most frequent mediastinal lymphadenopathy, configures Scadding I stage and is part of Scadding II stage. Right paratracheal and aortopulmonary locations are commonly observed on chest computed tomography (CT) and calcifications of lymph nodes may also occur [9].

2.2 Extrapulmonary sarcoidosis

After lung and mediastinal/hilar lymphadenopathy, skin, eye and joint are the most common sites of tissue affection [1].

2.2.1 Peripheral lymphadenopathy

More than 20% of patients have peripheral lymphadenopathy (cervical, axillary, inguinal and epitrochlear). The affected lymph nodes are moderately swollen and are usually painless [9].

2.2.2 Abdominal sarcoidosis

Sarcoidosis of the gastrointestinal (GI) tract is extremely rare: esophageal involvement in sarcoidosis may manifest as dysphagia and weight loss; the stomach, particularly the antrum, is the most frequently affected hollow organ in sarcoidosis.

The main symptom is postprandial epigastric pain and there may be early satiety, nausea, vomiting and weight loss. Ulcerations may cause upper GI bleeding and mucosal enlargements may cause antral narrowing, leading to gastric outlet obstruction; sarcoidosis of the small bowel is the least common form of GI sarcoidosis. Patients present with diarrhea, malabsorption, protein-losing enteropathy, periumbilical or epigastric pain, or hemorrhage. There may be associated folate deficiency or malabsorption of vitamin B12 with terminal ileal disease or achlorhydria; colonic sarcoidosis presents as multiple nodules, polyps, stenosis, obstructive lesions, aphthous erosions or small punctuate bleeding sites. Symptoms include abdominal pain in over 50% of cases [4].

Liver is a frequently affected site in sarcoidosis. It occurs in 20 to 30% of cases and is rarely severe [4]. However, a cluster of patients may develop severe complications such as cirrhosis and portal hypertension [10]. Jaundice is a rare symptom of liver disease, with pruritus and abdominal pain being seen more often; fever, although seldom a predominant feature, may be more common in patients with hepatic affection. Up to 35% of patients with sarcoidosis have abnormal liver function tests but these liver function tests are unrelated to the degree of aggression and extent of disease. Hepatomegaly can be found clinically and on abdominal computed tomography (CT) scan [4].

The spleen is enlarged on physical examination in 5–14% of patients with sarcoidosis. Involvement of the spleen causes symptoms in 15% of patients and is associated with hypersplenism in 20% of cases, most of whom have giant splenomegaly. In the majority of patients with splenomegaly, hepatomegaly and abnormal liver function tests are performed. Patients may develop splenic nodules and those patients with splenic nodules or hepatosplenomegaly are more likely to have symptoms than those without these findings [4]. Diffuse spleen involvement is a significant risk factor for a severe prognostic outcome in sarcoidosis [11].

Peritoneal sarcoidosis is a very rare disease whose symptoms include abdominal pain and ascites [12]. The clinical course of sarcoid-induced ascites not associated with portal hypertension is benign, with the condition resolving in the majority of patients. However, chylous ascites may develop because of obstruction of mesenteric lymphatics by sarcoid lymphadenopathy or by a fibrotic process [4].

Symptomatic pancreatic involvement usually occurs due to parenchymal disease or duct obstruction. Symptoms include abdominal pain, weight loss, jaundice, nausea and anorexia; and findings include a mass, usually in the head or a diffusely firm, nodular pancreas [4].

Acute cholecystitis as a complication of sarcoidosis may occur because of extrinsic compression of the cystic duct by granulomatous lymph nodes or by granulomatous inflammation of the gallbladder; obstructive jaundice may be due to granulomatous involvement of the common hepatic duct and surrounding lymph nodes; subacute or chronic cholecystitis with granulomas in the gallbladder wall is also described; chronic cholestasis related to cholangitis or extrahepatic bile duct involvement with typical findings of pruritis and jaundice has been reported less frequently [4].

Abdominal adenopathy is characterized by an increased number of normal-sized nodes, generally less than 2 cm in diameter. The nodes are most commonly found in the porta hepatis and less commonly involve the retrocrural area [6].

Renal sarcoidosis is likely underreported but isolated renal forms of sarcoidosis without extrarenal manifestations have been described. Renal involvement of sarcoidosis represents a relevant organ manifestation including granulomatous tubulointerstitial nephritis (the most typical form of renal sarcoidosis), secondary forms of glomerulonephritis and disorders in calcium homeostasis that can lead to nephrocalcinosis and nephrolithiasis. Renal masses and amyloid A (AA) amyloidosis are considered rare manifestations. There is a marked renal impairment [6].

2.2.3 Neurological sarcoidosis

Sarcoidosis affects the nervous system in 10% of cases [3] and approximately 5–7% of patients with systemic sarcoidosis [13] manifest symptoms of central or peripheral nervous system involvement, the so-called neurosarcoidosis (NS) [14]. Patients affected by sarcoidosis may also have subclinical neurological involvement in up to 26% of cases [13]. It can affect any part of the nervous system with all degrees of severity and may be very difficult to diagnose without histological confirmation [3]. NS may manifest as:

2.2.3.1 Cranial neuropathy (CN)

Cranial neuropathy is the most prevalent symptom of NS [13]. Within CN, facial nerve is the most affected, as it accounts for 70% of isolated CN. Most of the symptoms are unilateral and occur at the onset of disease [3].

Optic neuropathy is also common. A subacute optic neuritis is the most common presentation and it presents in an identical way to a demyelinating optic neuritis with pain being less prevalent, and the nadir acuity slightly less [3]. Synchronous bilateral optic neuritis is uncommon, but sequential optic neuropathies occurred in 30% in one study, and the same study showed 36% of concurrent intraocular inflammation development [15]. The associated field defects are central, centrocecal or altitudinal. An optic perineuritis can occur and lead to visual field constriction, disk swelling and pain. Chiasmal involvement is common when a basal leptomeningitis involves the hypothalamus and adjacent structures. Finally, a compressive optic neuropathy may arise when a dural inflammatory mass, usually at the orbital apex, involves the optic nerve. There may also be sensory loss and pain [3].

Isolated CN other than optic and facial are less common: the oculomotor, trochlear and abducens are relatively frequently involved, the trigeminal often alongside other nerves [16] (inflammatory masses within the orbit, at the orbital apex and cavernous sinus or spread from an adjacent basal leptomeningitis may cause diplopia, trigeminal sensory loss and pain, and proptosis [3]). The vestibulocochlear nerve is less frequently affected [16]. In fact, eighth nerve involvement is found in 1–7% of NS patients. Isolated hearing loss is uncommon in sarcoidosis. It occurs suddenly, often alongside a vestibular syndrome [13]. Spread from mastoid sinuses into the middle ear may also occur and the vestibulocochlear nerve may be involved as part of a spreading pachymeningitis or a leptomeningitis, often with accompanying facial nerve palsy. Isolated CN of the lowest cranial nerves are uncommon, but a bulbar disorder characterized by progressive dysphonia and dysphagia has been seen. Occasionally, there is weakness and atrophy of one side of the tongue. Involvement of these nerves may also form part of a more widespread disorder due to a basal meningitis [3].

2.2.3.2 Peripheral neuropathy

Peripheral neuropathy, not associated with concomitant central neurological disease, is uncommon in sarcoidosis, accounting for <5% of all cases. Symptoms are sensorimotor or purely sensory and they may manifest as mononeuritis multiplex, asymmetric neuropathy and mononeuropathies, particularly of the radial and ulnar nerves. Thoracic radiculopathy appears to be exclusive to sarcoidosis, presenting as burning numbness of the chest wall. Rarely, acute inflammatory demyelinating polyradiculoneuropathy can occur [3]. However, small fiber neuropathy is a common complication of sarcoidosis [17]. It is associated with a severe and very poor treatment responsive to distal neuropathic pain [3], somatic paresthesia and/or dysautonomia [17].

2.2.3.3 Pituitary and hypothalamic involvement

Prevalence of hypothalamic-pituitary (HP) involvement is estimated at 2.5% in patients with NS, which may lead to pituitary hormone abnormalities. Central hypogonadism occurred most frequently in a case series, followed by hypothyroidism, low insulin-like growth factor 1 (IGF-1) and corticoadrenal insufficiency. Diabetes insipidus was frequent (66%), but primary polydipsia leading to hyponatremia had also been reported. Primary polydipsia as well as obesity and behavioral changes are a reflection of hypothalamic involvement by NS and may contribute to some of the metabolic changes observed in these patients [14]. Hypogonadism was also the most frequently reported endocrine disorder in HP sarcoidosis in a multicenter study, followed by thyroid-stimulating hormone (TSH) deficiency, diabetes insipidus, hyperprolactinemia, adrenocorticotropic hormone (ACTH) deficiency and growth hormone (GH) deficiency (GHD). Panhypopituitarism had also been described [18]. At last, optic neuropathy may occur in HP NS due to mass effect or direct involvement of the optic chiasm [14].

2.2.3.4 Involvement of the brain

Involvement of the brain can be observed to take place through a pachymeningitis, a leptomeningitis and a vasculitis [3].

Pachymeningitis: Patients present with headache and focal neurological signs, often with seizures. If the cavernous sinus and orbital apex are involved, patients may present with pain, diplopia and optic neuropathy [16].

Leptomeningitis: In a prospective study, 75% of cases showed features of an invasive and destructive meningoencephalitis. Two-thirds presented with signs of diencephalic dysfunction and hydrocephalus, while a third had signs of involvement of the brainstem, with associated hydrocephalus. The disease course is subacute but increasingly rapid, and these patients are more disabled than those with a pachymeningitis (the two processes do not seem to overlap) [16].

Vasculitis: Vascular involvement does occur but it rarely has a direct clinical consequence [16]. Vascular involvement may be as infarction due to large vessel occlusion occurring without prelude [3], a crescendo series of transient ischemic attacks culminating in infarction [19] or by raised intracranial pressure and transient neurological deficits [20]. Intracranial hemorrhage (ICH) in NS is rare, probably as uncommon as cerebral infarction. According to a systematic literature review, 20% of patients had no prodromal symptoms before ICH, one-third of patients had one or a combination of prodromal symptoms for days to months: mostly new or worsening headaches, in some cases ataxia or cognitive difficulties and rarely daytime somnolence or seizures. At presentation, most patients had worsening or acute severe headache or seizures, some patients had acute posterior fossa syndrome and two patients presented with coma [21]. The hemorrhage is mostly supratentorial, followed by infratentorial and less frequently subarachnoid [8]. There may be multiple simultaneous intracerebral hematomas or a single intracerebral hematoma [22] and an intramedullary spinal cord hemorrhage was also described [23].

2.2.3.5 Spinal cord and cauda equina involvement

Although less common than in leptomeningeal and pachymeningeal forms of the condition, isolated disease of the spinal cord and cauda equina does occur. Most symptoms present with a subacute spinal cord lesion, in which there is a single cervical or thoracic longitudinally extensive lesion. Half of those with lower dorsal lesions also have cauda equina lesion whose signs are early sphincter disturbance and a predominantly sensory disorder; it is rarely painful. However, a motor disorder comprising a single motor root usually is painful. When there is an accompanying amyotrophy due to root involvement, it may be difficult to distinguish it from a motor neuron disease. A progressive cord lesion is less common [3].

2.2.3.6 Clinically isolated NS

Patients may present with neurological symptoms consistent with NS with no clear evidence of systemic sarcoidosis [19]. From those symptoms, systemic disease might or not be found and can even develop later [3].

2.2.4 Musculoskeletal sarcoidosis

Musculoskeletal manifestations of sarcoidosis occur in one-quarter to one-third of sarcoidosis patients [24] and can take place in multiple forms: bone involvement, sarcoid arthropathy and sarcoid myopathy [9].

Bone sarcoidosis is usually asymptomatic and its lesions are more often cystic than sclerotic or lytic. Bone involvement is often accompanied by overlying skin disease and is reported most frequently in the proximal and middle phalanges. Skull, nasal bones, maxilla, sternum, ribs, vertebra, pelvis, tibia and femur may also be affected. Spinal lesions may appear lytic, sclerotic or both and can involve any segment of the spine but spinal involvement is often asymptomatic [24].

The most common manifestation is sarcoid arthropathy [9] in the form of an acute arthritis that occurs as part of Löfgren's syndrome (LS). The ankles are the most frequently involved joint, bilateral in the majority of patients. Joint involvement can extend to other sites including the knees, wrists, elbows and metacarpophalangeal joints. Tenosynovitis and periarticular swelling are more common than true synovitis. Chronic sarcoid arthritis is characterized by symmetric, medium to large joint oligoarthritis [24] and is usually associated with extra-articular sarcoidosis [9]. Destructive arthritis is less frequently described and there are case reports of sarcoid monoarthritis, although it is rare. Jaccoud's arthritis has been described in case reports and it usually presents in the context of extensive internal organ involvement later during the disease course. Dactylitis is almost exclusively associated with chronic systemic involvement and is a common form of musculoskeletal involvement. It is associated with swelling and erythema and typically develops in a symmetrical pattern, most often affecting the second and third phalanges, preserving the metacarpophalangeal joints [24].

Skeletal muscle involvement occurs in as many as half of all sarcoidosis patients [25]. Asymptomatic granulomatous muscle involvement in sarcoidosis is more common than symptomatic one. Muscle involvement includes a nodular type, an acute sarcoid myopathy type and a chronic sarcoid myopathy type (the most frequent type of sarcoid myopathy [25]) [24]. The main symptom is weakness, followed by myalgia [25] and reduced exercise capacity [24]. Nodular sarcoid myopathy is characterized by symmetrical limb involvement with single or multiple nodules in the muscles [24] that may cause pain and stiffness with cramps [25]. Acute myopathy is the least common form of sarcoid myopathy. It occurs early in the course of sarcoidosis and in patients <40 years of age. It presents with rapid onset of proximal weakness and myalgia associated with elevated creatinine kinase levels. Chronic sarcoid myopathy is reported in female patients between the ages of 50 and 60 years [24]. It is a slowly progressive symmetrical disease involving the proximal muscles of the extremities, trunk and neck, often with muscle wasting [25].

2.2.5 Ocular sarcoidosis

Ocular involvement manifests in 25–60% of patients with systemic sarcoidosis in two peaks of incidence, the first at 20–30 years and the second at 50–60 years [26]. Any structure within the eye may be involved, but uveitis is the most frequent form of ocular manifestation and may affect up to 20–30% of patients with sarcoidosis [9]. After uveitis, the most frequent feature is conjunctival involvement. Lacrimal gland or conjunctival involvement is usually asymptomatic, although extensive granulomas leading to diplopia or severe keratoconjunctivitis sicca may develop. Eyelid granulomas were repeatedly reported while corneal involvement by granulomas is extremely rare [26]; orbital symptoms mimic other inflammatory syndromes manifesting in the orbit (diffuse orbital inflammation, usually unilateral, which can result in ptosis, limitations of ocular movements and diplopia [27]). At scleral level, there may be scleritis or episcleritis and sarcoid-induced inflammatory myositis may resemble Graves' ophthalmopathy [26].

Acute signs of uveitis as pain, photophobia, lacrimation or redness might be absent, so that the patients with sarcoid-associated "silent uveitis" may develop permanent ocular damage before the intraocular process is diagnosed and treatment initiated [26]. Sarcoid uveitis is generally bilateral with the same findings and clinical course in both eyes [28]. Anterior uveitis is the most common anatomical form of intraocular inflammation, followed by posterior uveitis, intermediate uveitis and panuveitis [9]. Classic sarcoid-associated anterior uveitis may either present as an acute self-limiting [29] iridocyclitis or as a chronic granulomatous uveitis with keratic precipitates. Chronic anterior uveitis may lead to secondary cataract, glaucoma and cystoid macular edema. Intermediate uveitis with vitritis and genuine snow banking may be occasionally encountered but more frequent is the presence of vitritis with peripheral vasculitis and snowball infiltrates. This type of intermediate uveitis may precede more severe posterior segment changes [26]. Characteristic findings of posterior uveitis include retinal periphlebitis associated with segmental cuffing, extensive sheathing and perivenous infiltrates, referred to as "candle-wax drippings" [28]. The association of posterior segment and neurological involvement in sarcoidosis has been reported to be as high as 27%. The most frequent complications of posterior segment involvement in sarcoidosis include cystoid macular edema, cataract, glaucoma, retinal ischemia and neovascularizations. Poor visual prognosis is associated with advanced age, African-American ethnicity, female sex, chronic systemic disease and also with posterior segment involvement, the presence of cystoid macular edema and glaucoma [26].

DOI: http://dx.doi.org/10.5772/intechopen.1002282

2.2.6 Cardiac sarcoidosis

Cardiac involvement affects approximately 3 to 39% of patients with systemic sarcoidosis [9]. The cardiovascular involvement is usually associated with a bad prognosis. The most frequent clinical symptoms are palpitations, lipothymia and syncope. Among all arrhythmias, the most represented are those secondary to alterations of the conduction pathways (atrioventricular node, bundle of His and intraventricular pathways) which can progress toward a complete atrioventricular block that can lead to clinical symptoms such as syncope, sudden death and also to ventricular tachyarrhythmias. Atrioventricular block is the most common clinical manifestation of disease onset followed by ventricular tachyarrhythmias. Supraventricular tachyarrhythmias have a prevalence three times greater in cardiac sarcoidosis than in sarcoidosis patients without cardiac involvement and the most frequent supraventricular tachyarrhythmia is atrial fibrillation, followed by atrial tachycardia and atrial flutter [30].

Heart failure is an onset manifestation of the disease in 16% of cases, less frequently than arrhythmias. However, it is the second cause of death, only after sudden death from ventricular arrhythmias. Asthenia, dyspnea and orthopnea are related to heart failure, and the involvement of the ventricle can lead to the onset of cardiomyopathy at a young age. Patients with sarcoidosis also have an increased risk of cardiovascular events compared to the control population [30].

2.2.7 Cutaneous sarcoidosis

Cutaneous sarcoidosis is the initial manifestation of the disease in nearly one-third of patients. The skin is most often involved in African Americans [8].

Specific sarcoidosis lesions have granulomas on histological examination and apple-jelly coloration characteristic of granulomatous skin lesions on diascopy. Depending on the skin color, specific lesions range from flesh tinted to brown, to pink or violaceous. Specific sarcoidosis lesions include maculopapular sarcoidosis (lesions not only on the face, especially on the nasal folds, eyelids and orbits but also on the nape of neck, back, buttocks and extremities); the very common papular sarcoidosis (discrete papules measuring ≤1 cm that are commonly present on the face, especially around the eyelids and nasolabial folds. Papules can coalesce into plaques, are often associated with minimal to no systemic disease and may resolve spontaneously); the very common plaque sarcoidosis (single or multiple round, oval or annular plaques on the face, back, buttocks and extensor surface of the extremities. The plaques are thick and indurated and often heal with scarring or pigmentary changes); the common lupus pernio (reddish purple to violaceous brown, shiny, indurated plaques frequently over the central face, especially on the nasal alae, cheeks, lips and ears, and rarely on dorsal face of hands and feet. Lupus pernio lesions, predominantly occurring in African Americans, enlarge and are progressively disfiguring, causing nasal ulceration, septal perforation and obstruction); the common subcutaneous sarcoidosis (single to multiple asymptomatic to mildly tender, indurated skin-colored, panniculitic plaques or nodules characteristically on the extremities, particularly the forearms); the common scar sarcoidosis (granulomatous infiltration of surgical scars, tattoos, skin piercings and other sites of trauma); the common nodular sarcoidosis; and other uncommon or rare specific lesions of cutaneous sarcoidosis like annular, angiolupoid, verrucous, lichenoid, psoriasiform, hypopigmented, atrophic, ulcerative, ichthyosiform, erythrodermic, morpheaform, photodistributed, sarcoidal alopecia, oral, genital and nail sarcoidosis [8].

Nonspecific sarcoidosis skin lesions lack granulomas and are caused by inflammatory reactions to sarcoidosis. Erythema nodosum (EN) is the most common nonspecific sarcoidosis skin manifestation, occurring in 10% of patients [8]. EN is a form of panniculitis (inflammatory processes that affect the subcutaneous cellular tissue) characterized by tender erythematous nodules mainly in the lower limbs on the pretibial area [31]. On histology, lesions show a septal panniculitis without granulomas [8]. EN is considered a hypersensitivity response to a variety of antigenic stimuli which can be infections, inflammation, neoplastic disease, pregnancy and/or drugs [31]. Other nonspecific manifestations of sarcoidosis include Sweet syndrome, erythema multiforme, pyoderma gangrenosum, prurigo, calcinosis cutis, vasculitis and digital clubbing [8]. All these nonspecific skin manifestations (EN included) can be a skin manifestation of a non-sarcoidosis disease and so, although they can be associated with sarcoidosis, their presence does not mean cutaneous sarcoidosis.

Although most lesions have distinct features that allow recognition or at least enable a high level of suspicion, sarcoidosis skin manifestations can mimic nearly any skin disease [8]. Some patterns of cutaneous involvement may be associated with specific extracutaneous manifestations of sarcoidosis, while other patterns may predict systemic disease severity and response to treatment [9].

2.2.8 Head and neck sarcoidosis

Multiple manifestations are possible in the head and neck region (HNR), such as lymphadenitis colli, acute or chronic sinusitis and swelling of the parotid glands, as part of Heerfordt's syndrome or xerostomia. The clinical findings are often nonspecific. The most frequent manifestation of sarcoidosis in the HNR is cervical lymphadenopathy, followed by nose or parasinusal affection, cervical skin or parotid gland affection [32]. Larynx is the less frequently involved organ in the HNR [9]. While the major salivary gland involvement most frequently follows a benign course, sinonasal and laryngeal sarcoidosis are usually severe [9]. Patients with sinonasal disease have nonspecific upper respiratory symptoms like nasal obstruction, rhinorrhea, anosmia, crusting rhinitis, epistaxis and facial pain [33]. Laryngeal sarcoidosis usually involves the supraglottis (epiglottis, then arytenoids) and does not affect the vocal cords [9]. The symptoms range from hoarseness, inspiratory dyspnea, dysphagia, chronic cough and obstructive sleep apnea to airway obstruction requiring a tracheotomy [33].

2.2.9 Bone marrow sarcoidosis

Bone marrow involvement is a rare extrapulmonary sarcoidosis tissue affection. It is present in approximately 6% of cases of pulmonary sarcoidosis [34], but isolated sarcoidosis of the marrow as an initial presentation, without involvement of other organ systems, is not as common [35].

Although peripheral blood tests may show evidence of anemia, leukopenia or lymphopenia [35], bone marrow involvement can present with normal hematological parameters [36].

2.3 Clinical phenotypes and clinical syndromes

Multiple manifestations and associations of organ involvement occur to configure clinical phenotypes/syndromes.

2.3.1 Clinical phenotypes

A European multicenter study [1] identified five distinct phenotypes based on predominant organ involvement and organ manifestations that frequently occur together:

Cluster (1) Abdominal organ involvement (liver, spleen, kidney): in patients with liver involvement, there was often spleen, kidney and intrathoracic lymph node involvement. These patients experienced weight loss, night sweats and presented significantly more often with impaired lung function.

Cluster (2) Ocular-cardiac-cutaneous-central nervous system (CNS) disease involvement (eye/heart/skin/salivary glands/CNS): In cardiac and skin sarcoidosis, fatigue and arthralgia were more prevalent than in patients without these organ manifestations. In patients with eye involvement, there was also a higher rate of arthralgia but a reduced frequency of fever. In NS, fatigue was also more prevalent.

Cluster (3) Musculoskeletal-cutaneous involvement: patients with arthritis or musculoskeletal involvement presented significantly more often with an acute onset and suffered more from fever, night sweats, weight loss and arthralgia. These patients showed more often involvement of the skin, intrathoracic lymph nodes and kidneys but less often of the lungs or bronchi. Patients with musculoskeletal sarcoidosis also suffered significantly more often from eye involvement.

Cluster (4) Pulmonary and intrathoracic lymph node involvement: patients with lung involvement had worse lung function and presented more often with dyspnea, cough, chest pain and fatigue. These patients suffered more often from bronchial and intrathoracic lymph node involvement, but less often from skin or musculoskeletal involvement.

Cluster (5) Extrapulmonary involvement: the extrapulmonary phenotype had the highest frequency of kidney involvement.

These phenotypes are only applicable in Caucasian cohorts and might be different in African or Asian populations [1].

Another cohort study [37] identified six discrete phenotypes of sarcoidosis: C1 (pure LS with BHL and erythema nodosum), C2 (febrile LS), C3 (nonfebrile LS with periarticular ankle inflammation), C4 (exclusive pulmonary sarcoidosis), C5 (pulmonary sarcoidosis and abdominal involvement) and C6 (organ involvement different from the lungs, including: skin lesions, peripheral lymph nodes and neurological and ocular involvement).

Lastly, a multicenter study [38] identified five clinical phenotypes of extrapulmonary sarcoidosis: (1) erythema nodosum, joint involvement and hilar lymph nodes, mainly in European/Caucasian female patients; (2) neurological, digestive and/or kidney involvement; (3) parenchymal lung involvement and fibrosis, cardiac and skin involvement, mainly in non-European/Caucasian patients; (4) lupus pernio and severe involvement; and (5) parenchymal pulmonary involvement, peripheral nodes, and hepatic, splenic and bone involvement, mainly in non-European/Caucasian patients. This study also identified a preferential association of organ involvement: erythema nodosum with joint involvement; hepatic, splenic, bone and peripheral node involvement; pulmonary with cardiac involvement; kidney with digestive involvement; lupus pernio with ear, nose and throat involvement; and uveitis with neurological involvement [38].

2.3.2 Clinical syndromes

Löfgren's syndrome is a well-differentiated form of sarcoidosis with characteristic epidemiological, clinical, radiological and prognostic features. LS is the triad of bilateral hilar lymphadenopathy with erythema nodosum and/or articular involvement (usually periarticular ankle inflammation) and/or fever. Patients typically experience an acute onset of the disease, is more frequent in females and it usually occurs between the age of 25 and 40 years, with a second peak around the age of 45 to 60 years [39]. The different manifestations of LS differ according to sex: EN is found predominantly in women while arthropathy/arthritis is more common in men [9]. Other extrapulmonary manifestations were observed in a cohort of patients with LS: granulomatous skin lesions, hepatomegaly, ocular involvement, splenomegaly, salivary gland hypertrophy and CNS involvement. LS is usually a self-limiting disease but some patients develop chronic disease [40].

Heerfordt-Waldenström's syndrome, also called uveoparotid fever as it is associated with low-grade fever [9], comprises a granulomatous uveitis, parotid and submandibular salivary gland swelling and cranial neuropathy (usually but not always the facial nerve) [3]. LS and Heerfordt's syndrome are considered to be highly specific of the disease and do not require histological confirmation [9].

3. Conclusion

Sarcoidosis is a granulomatous disease of unknown etiology that is characterized by the development of granulomatous inflammation in affected tissues. Any tissue can be affected and the same organ involvement may be presented in multiple ways. Also, sarcoidosis may be asymptomatic or cause a symptomatic multisystem disease. To add on to the variability of clinical presentation, clinical manifestations vary with race, sex, age and type of disease onset. Female patients are globally more affected. Clinical onset may be acute or subacute and clinical course self-remitting or chronic.

The most common manifestation is pulmonary sarcoidosis, followed by skin, eye and joint involvement. Respiratory and cardiac sarcoidosis contribute to the greater mortality rate associated with sarcoidosis compared to the general population and these patients also have more other morbidities.

It is important to be aware of sarcoidosis' wide range of manifestations in order to achieve diagnosis so that patients can be followed and treated.

Acknowledgements

No funding was received for the development of this paper.

Conflict of interest

The authors declare no conflict of interest.

Author details

Inês S.F. da Silva*, Ryan Costa Silva, Inês Sopa and Lígia Peixoto
Hospital de Santa Maria, Centro Hospitalar Universitario Lisboa Norte, Lisbon, Portugal

*Address all correspondence to: ines.s.silva81@gmail.com

References

[1] Schupp JC, Freitag-Wolf S, Bargagli E, Mihailović-Vučinić V, Rottoli P, Grubanovic A, et al. Phenotypes of organ involvement in sarcoidosis. European Respiratory Journal. 2018;**51**(1):1700991

[2] Mañá J, Rubio-Rivas M, Villalba N, Marcoval J, Iriarte A, Molina-Molina M, et al. Multidisciplinary approach and long-term follow-up in a series of 640 consecutive patients with sarcoidosis. Medicine. 2017;**96**(29):e7595

[3] Kidd DP. Neurosarcoidosis: Clinical manifestations, investigation and treatment. Practical Neurology. 2020;**20**(3):199-212

[4] Ebert EC, Kierson M, Hagspiel KD. Gastrointestinal and hepatic manifestations of sarcoidosis. American Journal of Gastroenterology. 2008;**103**(12):3184-3192

[5] Baughman RP, Teirstein AS, Judson MA, Rossman MD, Yeager H, Bresnitz EA, et al. Clinical characteristics of patients in a case control study of sarcoidosis. American Journal of Respiratory and Critical Care Medicine. 2001;**164**(10 Pt 1):1885-1889

[6] Bergner R, Löffler C. Renal sarcoidosis: Approach to diagnosis and management. Current Opinion in Pulmonary Medicine. 2018;**24**(5):513-520

[7] Jamilloux Y, Bonnefoy M, Valeyre D, Varron L, Broussolle C, Sève P. Elderly-onset sarcoidosis: Prevalence, clinical course, and treatment. Drugs and Aging. 2013;**30**(12):969-978

[8] Sanchez M, Haimovic A, Prystowsky S. Sarcoidosis. Dermatologic Clinics. 2015;**33**(3):389-416

[9] Sève P, Pacheco Y, Durupt F, Jamilloux Y, Gerfaud-Valentin M, Isaac S, et al. Sarcoidosis: A clinical overview from symptoms to diagnosis. Cell. 2021;**10**(4):766-799

[10] Rossi G, Ziol M, Roulot D, Valeyre D, Mahévas M. Hepatic sarcoidosis: Current concepts and treatments. Seminars in Respiratory and Critical Care Medicine. 2020;**41**(5):652-658

[11] Tetikkurt C, Yanardag H, Pehlivan M, Bilir M. Clinical features and prognostic significance of splenic involvement in sarcoidosis. Monaldi Archives for Chest Disease. 2017;**87**(3):135-139

[12] Roh WS, Lee S, Park JH, Kang J. Abdominal sarcoidosis mimicking peritoneal carcinomatosis. Annals of Coloproctology. 2018;**34**(2):101-105

[13] Cama E, Santarelli R, Muzzi E, Inches I, Curtolo S, Di Paola F, et al. Sudden hearing loss in sarcoidosis: Otoneurological study and neuroradiological correlates Ipoacusia improvvisa nella sarcoidosi: studio otoneurologico e riscontri neuroradiologici. Acta Otorhinolaryngologica Italica. 2011;**31**(4):235-238

[14] Anthony J, Esper GJ, Ioachimescu A. Hypothalamic–pituitary sarcoidosis with vision loss and hypopituitarism: case series and literature review. Pituitary. 2016;**19**(1):19-29

[15] Kidd DP, Burton BJ, Graham EM, Plant GT. Optic neuropathy associated with systemic sarcoidosis. Neurology Neuroimmunology Neuroinflammation. 2016;**3**(5):e270

[16] Kidd DP. Sarcoidosis of the central nervous system: Clinical features,

imaging, and CSF results. Journal of Neurology. 2018;**265**(8):1906-1915

[17] Tavee JO, Karwa K, Ahmed Z, Thompson N, Parambil J, Culver DA. Sarcoidosis-associated small fiber neuropathy in a large cohort: Clinical aspects and response to IVIG and anti-TNF alpha treatment. Respiratory Medicine. 2017;**126**:135-138

[18] Langrand C, Bihan H, Raverot G, Varron L, Androdias G, Borson-Chazot F, et al. Hypothalamo-pituitary sarcoidosis: A multicenter study of 24 patients. QJM. 2012;**105**(10):981-995

[19] Brown MM, Thompson AJ, Wedzicha JA, Swash M. Sarcoidosis presenting with stroke. Stroke. 1989;**20**(3):400-405

[20] Campbell J, Kee R, Bhattacharya D, Flynn P, McCarron M, Fulton A. Systemic sarcoidosis presenting with headache and stroke-like episodes. Case Reports in Immunology. 2015;**2015**:1-5

[21] O'Dwyer JP, Al-Moyeed BA, Farrell MA, Pidgeon CN, Collins DR, Fahy A, et al. Neurosarcoidosis-related intracranial haemorrhage: Three new cases and a systematic review of the literature. European Journal of Neurology. 2013;**20**(1):71-78

[22] Vukojević Z, Ilić TV, Dominović-Kovačević A, Grgić S, Mavija S. Neurosarcoidosis and multiple intracerebral hematomas: An unusual clinical presentation. Journal of the Neurological Sciences. 2017;**379**:22-24

[23] Pegat B, Drapier S, Morandi X, Edan G. Spinal cord hemorrhage in a patient with neurosarcoidosis on long-term corticosteroid therapy: Case report. BMC Neurology. 2015;**15**(1):123-127

[24] Bechman K, Christidis D, Walsh S, Birring SS, Galloway J. A review of the musculoskeletal manifestations of sarcoidosis. Rheumatology (Oxford). 2018;**57**(5):777-783

[25] Wolfe SM, Pinals RS, Aelion JA, Goodman RE. Myopathy in sarcoidosis: Clinical and pathologic study of four cases and review of the literature. Seminars in Arthritis and Rheumatism. 1987;**16**(4):300-306

[26] Rothova A. Ocular involvement in sarcoidosis. British Journal of Ophthalmology. 2000;**84**(1):110-116

[27] Sève P, Jamilloux Y, Tilikete C, Gerfaud-Valentin M, Kodjikian L, El Jammal T. Ocular sarcoidosis. Seminars in Respiratory and Critical Care Medicine. 2020;**41**(5):673-688

[28] Jamilloux Y, Kodjikian L, Broussolle C, Sève P. Sarcoidosis and uveitis. Autoimmunity Reviews. 2014;**13**(8):840-849

[29] Ma SP, Rogers SL, Hall AJ, Hodgson L, Brennan J, Stawell RJ, et al. Sarcoidosis-related uveitis: Clinical presentation, disease course, and rates of systemic disease progression after uveitis diagnosis. American Journal of Ophthalmology. 2019;**198**:30-36

[30] Tana C, Mantini C, Donatiello I, Mucci L, Tana M, Ricci F, et al. Clinical features and diagnosis of cardiac sarcoidosis. Journal of Clinical Medicine. 2021;**10**(9):1941-1952

[31] Pérez-Garza DM, Chavez-Alvarez S, Ocampo-Candiani J, Gomez-Flores M. Erythema nodosum: A practical approach and diagnostic algorithm. American Journal of Clinical Dermatology. 2021;**22**(3):367-378

[32] Send T, Korsten P, Bertlich M, Braunwarth C, Bootz F, Skowasch D, et al. Clinical features of sarcoidosis patients presenting with head and

neck manifestations–a two-center retrospective study and proposal of a diagnostic algorithm for the otorhinolaryngologist. Acta Oto-Laryngologica. 2020;**140**(2):144-148

[33] Edriss H, Kelley JS, Demke J, Nugent K. Sinonasal and laryngeal sarcoidosis—An uncommon presentation and management challenge. American Journal of the Medical Sciences. 2019;**357**(2):93-102

[34] Brandão, Calçada M, Montezinho S, Teixeira AM, Gomes B, Macedo B. Sarcoidosis with rare extrapulmonary involvement. European Journal of Case Reports in Internal Medicine. 2021;**8**(7):002540

[35] Miller AC, Chacko T, Rashid RM, Ledford DK. Fever of unknown origin and isolated noncaseating granuloma of the marrow: Could this be sarcoidosis? Allergy and Asthma Proceedings. 2007;**28**(2):230-235

[36] Hameed OA, Skibinska M. Scar sarcoidosis with bone marrow involvement and associated musculoskeletal symptoms. BMJ Case Reports. 2011;**2011**:bcr0220113863

[37] Rubio-Rivas M, Corbella X. Clinical phenotypes and prediction of chronicity in sarcoidosis using cluster analysis in a prospective cohort of 694 patients. European Journal of Internal Medicine. 2020;**77**:59-65

[38] Lhote R, Annesi-Maesano I, Nunes H, Launay D, Borie R, Sacré K, et al. Clinical phenotypes of extrapulmonary sarcoidosis: An analysis of a French, multi-ethnic, multicentre cohort. European Respiratory Journal. 2021;**57**(4):2001160

[39] Rubio-Rivas M, Franco J, Corbella X. Sarcoidosis presenting with and without Löfgren's syndrome: Clinical, radiological and behavioral differences observed in a group of 691 patients. Joint Bone Spine. 2020;**87**(2):141-147

[40] Mañá J, Gómez-Vaquero C, Montero A, Salazar A, Marcoval J, Valverde J, et al. Löfgren's syndrome revisited: A study of 186 patients. The American Journal of Medicine. 1999;**107**(3):240-245

Chapter 3

Cutaneous Manifestations of Sarcoid: Clinical Presentation and Histopathology

Lily Lebwohl and Robert G. Phelps

Abstract

The cutaneous manifestations of sarcoid will be reviewed. These include lupus pernio, multiple varied skin presentations such as annular sarcoid, hyperpigmentation, hypopigmentation, erythroderma, scar-like lesions, and several others. Erythema nodosum in sarcoidosis will be discussed; the Koebner phenomenon will be described; and the differential diagnosis of all of these lesions will be presented in detail. Numerous clinical photographs will be provided to help the treating clinician identify and work up the patient accordingly. The histopathology and pathologic differential diagnosis will also be discussed. Treatments for the varied skin lesions will be reviewed in detail as will the side effects of each treatment and management overview.

Keywords: lupus pernio, cutaneous sarcoid, erythema nodosum, granulomatous, Koebner

1. Introduction

Sarcoid is a granulomatous disease that is known to affect multiple organ systems and primarily the lungs [1]. It can also affect the heart, kidneys, eyes, liver, joints, and lymph nodes [2–4]. The many clinical presentations of sarcoid has led to its being called the great imitator as many conditions are misdiagnosed as sarcoid and sarcoid is misdiagnosed as other diseases. The differential diagnosis must therefore conditions as varied as leishmaniasis, leprosy, infectious diseases, vasculitides, drug reactions, granulomatous reactions to environmental agents, lupus rheumatoid arthritis, ankylosing spondylitis, common variable immune deficiency, lymphomatoid granulomatosis, paracoccidioidomycosis and others [5–11].

The skin is commonly involved in sarcoid, affecting up to 30% of patients [12, 13].

Like the many systemic manifestations of sarcoid, the cutaneous manifestations are quite varied, and many of the cutaneous manifestations will be described below.

2. Epidemiology

Sarcoid can affect individuals of all ages, but primarily manifests in young adults. It displays heterogeneity and follows an unpredictable clinical trajectory [14].

IntechOpen

The frequency of sarcoid varies significantly across different parts of the world. In South Korea, Taiwan, and Japan, the occurrence ranges from 1 to 5 cases per 100,000 individuals, whereas in Sweden and Canada, rates of 140 to 160 cases per 100,000 people [15]. The skin is commonly affected [12] affecting up to 30% of patients [13]. There are familial cases as well [16]. Sarcoid is most commonly found in non-Hispanic Black individuals in the United States, particularly among Black American women who exhibit the highest occurrence and prevalence rates [17]. We present a review of the pathology of cutaneous sarcoid and numerous clinical cutaneous presentations with figures.

3. Cutaneous manifestations

There are many cutaneous presentations of sarcoid. The most characteristic lesions are papules and nodules on the face called lupus pernio (**Figure 1**). The nose

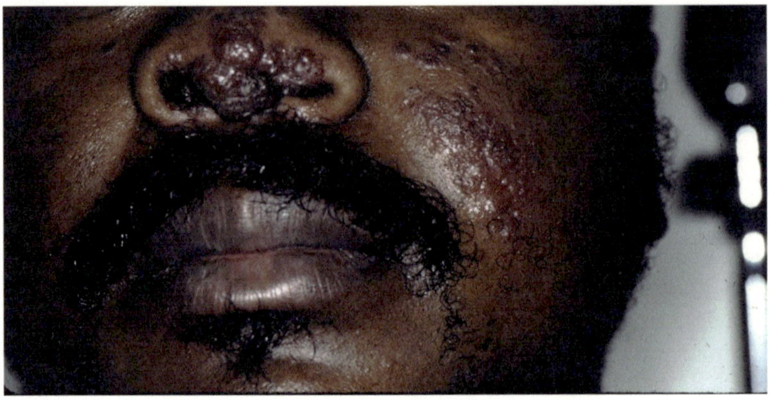

Figure 1.
Sarcoid, papules and nodules.

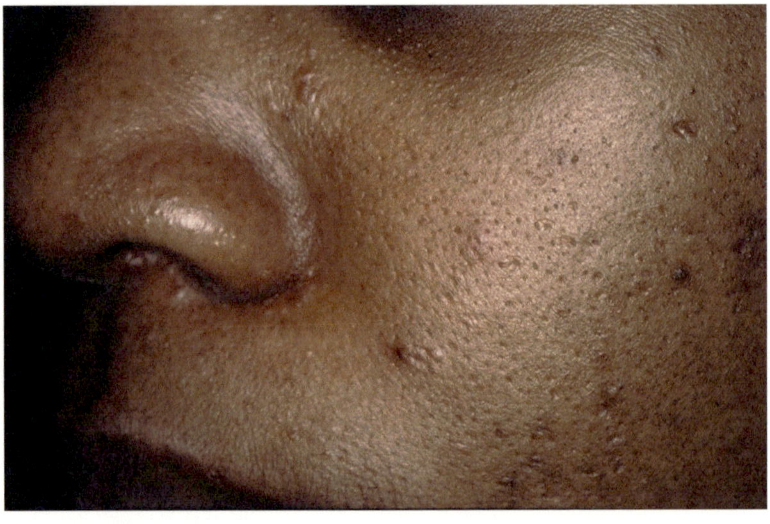

Figure 2.
KT pseudofolliculitis barbae-like sarcoid.

is prominently affected. It affects both African American and Caucasian patients. Papules can be found on the entrance to the nose (**Figure 2**) and on the ear (**Figure 3**). It can also occur around the lips and at the angle of the mouth (**Figure 4**). Lesions can

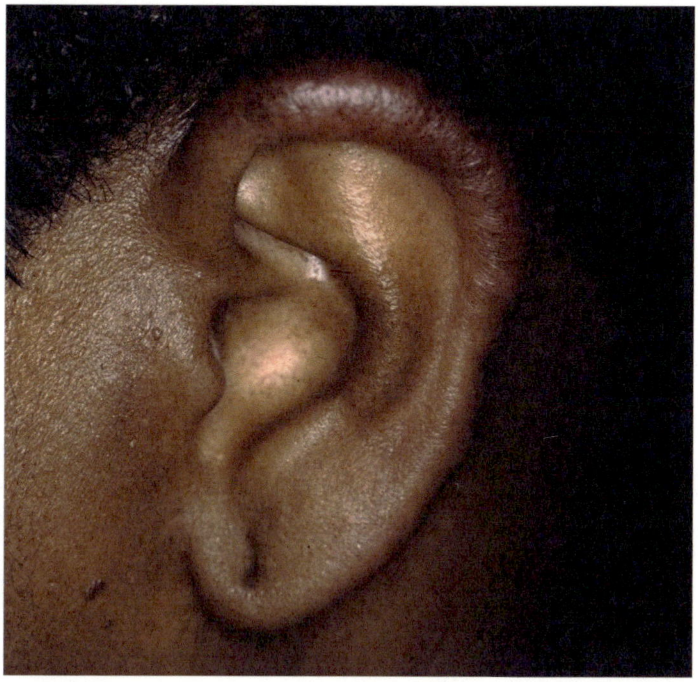

Figure 3.
Sarcoid FF.

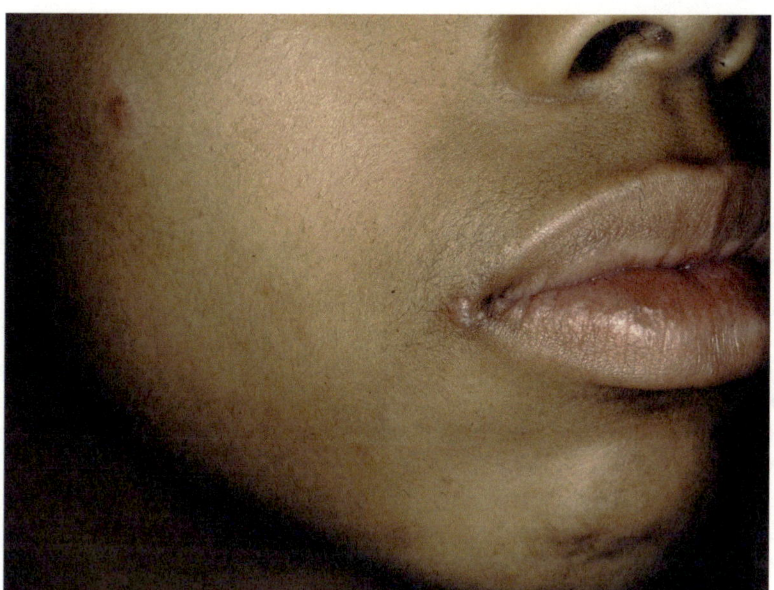

Figure 4.
Sarcoid, IT, lupus pernio papules at oral commissure.

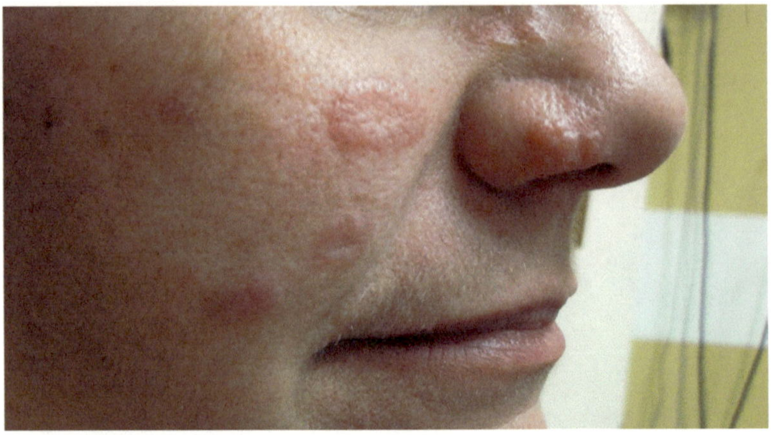

Figure 5.
Annular sarcoid lupus Pernio.

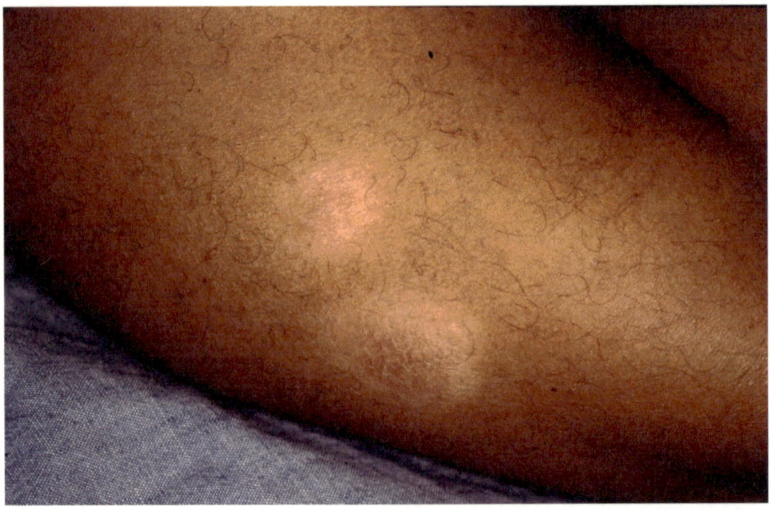

Figure 6.
Hypopigmented sarcoid.

be annular, (**Figure 5**) can appear hypopigmented (**Figure 6**), and hyperpigmented patches with papules (**Figure 7**) can also develop. The lesions of sarcoid can be scar-like and the scars can ulcerate (**Figure 8**) and can affect African American patients (**Figure 9**). Ulcerations are not rare in Caucasian or African American patients (**Figure 10**). Lesions can also be covered with telangiectasia and sarcoid can present with the Koebner phenomenon (**Figure 11**).

The condition can mimic numerous other cutaneous diseases including hypertrophic scars (**Figure 12**) and psoriasis (**Figure 13**). Another condition that sarcoid can simulate is pseudofolliculitis barbae (**Figure 14**), stasis dermatitis (**Figure 15**), and patients can develop enlarged noses resembling rhinophyma (**Figure 16**). Sarcoid can

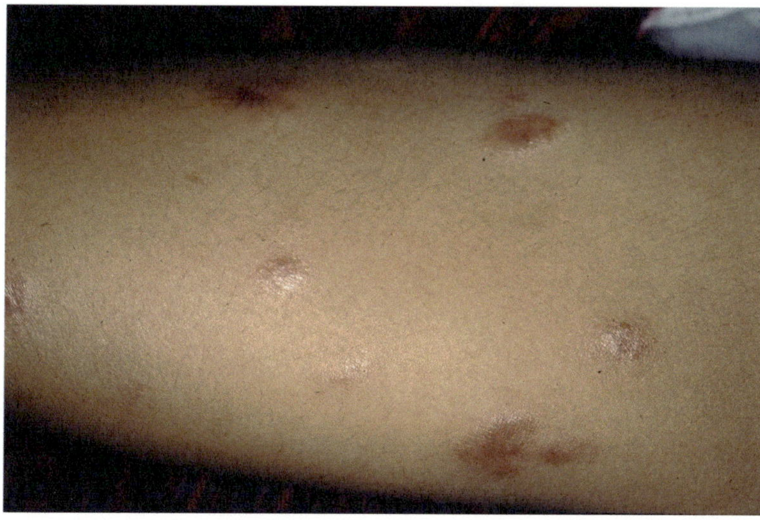

Figure 7.
IT scar like.

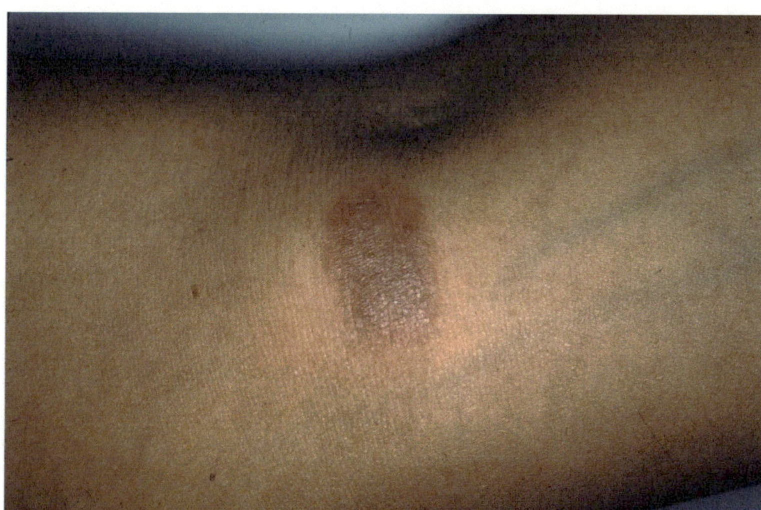

Figure 8.
Sarcoid, FA.

resemble acne nuchae keloidalis (**Figure 17**) and there are patients who present with clusters of brown papules resembling lichen nitidus (**Figure 18**). African American patients can be affected more severely (**Figures 19** and **20**) [18].

Erythema nodosum has occurred as a reaction to sarcoid. While there are many conditions that lead to erythema nodosum, sarcoid is classically one of them. When erythema nodosum occurs in sarcoid patients, it has been said to portend a good outcome to the sarcoid (**Figure 21**) [19] with resolution of the disease thereafter.

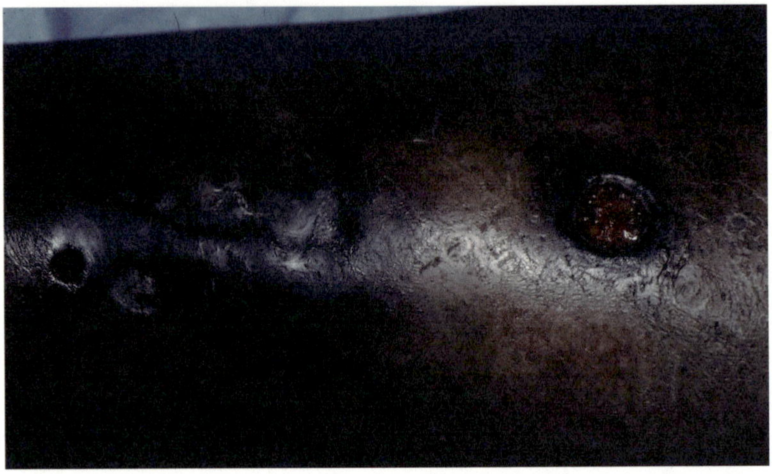

Figure 9.
Sarcoid, KS.

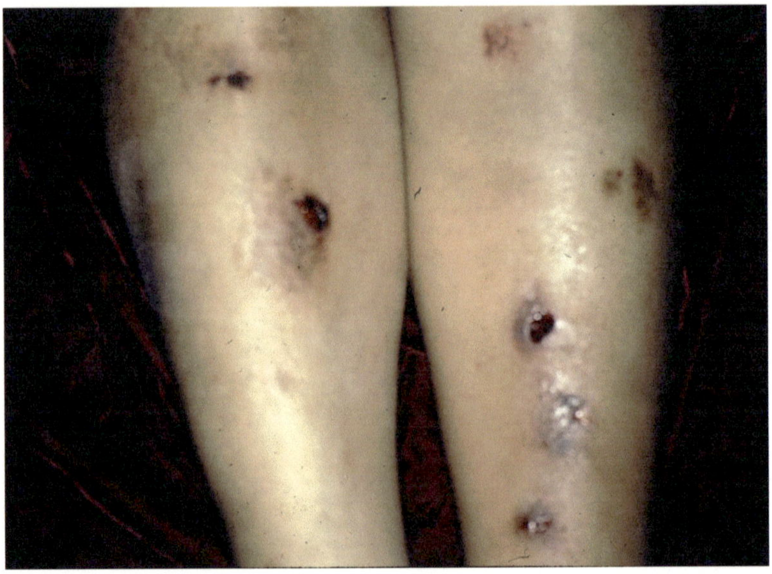

Figure 10.
Sarcoid, leg ulcers.

Skin lesions have been treated with all the therapies that have been used for sarcoid including systemic steroids, methotrexate, antimalarials, TNF blockers [20]. The patient shown in **Figure 22** was treated only with intralesional corticosteroids with complete resolution of her sarcoid (**Figure 23**).

4. Histopathology

Definitive diagnosis of cutaneous sarcoidosis will be determined by a skin biopsy to confirm the clinical impression. Although almost any type of biopsy will most

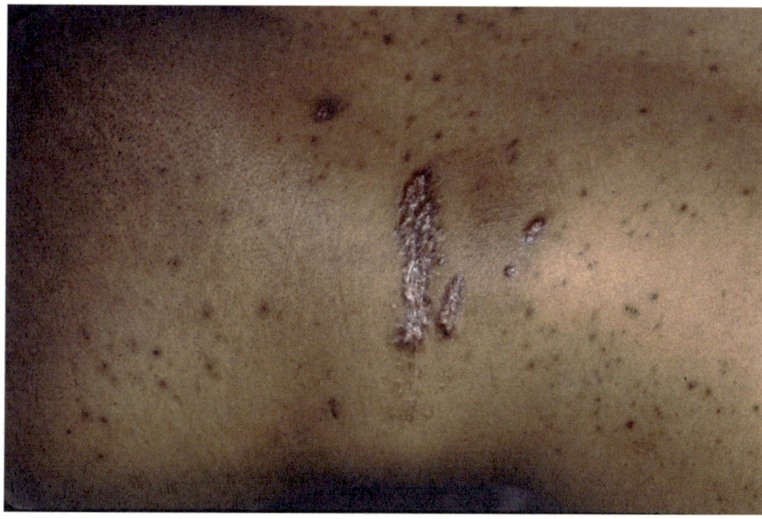

Figure 11.
Sarcoid, scarlike with Koebner phenomenon.

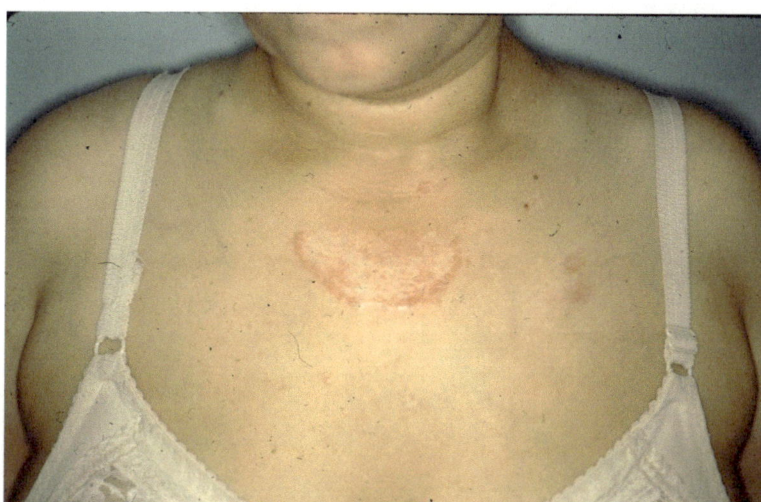

Figure 12.
Sarcoid, CS presterna; scar, annular.

likely yield an appropriate diagnosis, it imperative that the biopsy be representative. In most instances a 3 or 4 mm punch biopsy will yield enough information. However, sometimes sarcoidosis can be present in the subcutis and a deeper incisional biopsy will be necessary.

Fortunately, in most instances pathology has characteristic features. Throughout the superficial and deep dermis, there are nodular collections of epithelioid cells. The epithelioid cells have a distinctive appearance: oval histiocytes with abundant amphophilic or eosinophilic cytoplasm and eccentric angulated nuclei. At the periphery, frequently there are multinucleated giant cells arranged in horseshoe like shape "Langhans type giant cells" (**Figure 24**) Surrounding these granulomas, there is often

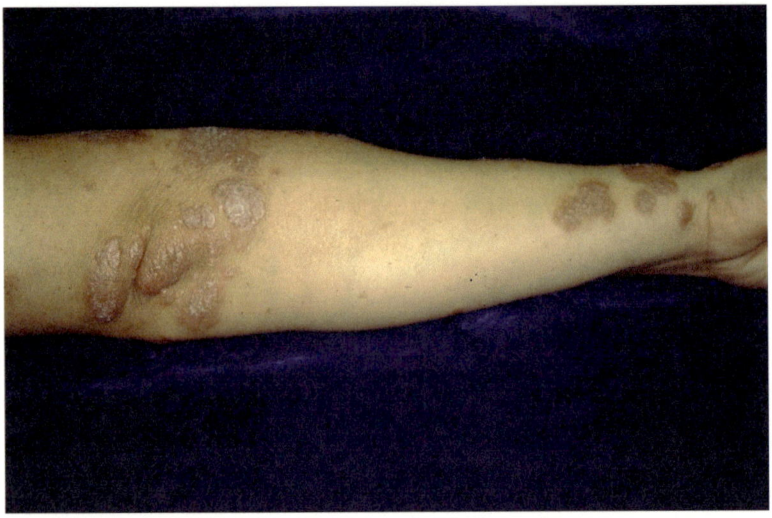

Figure 13.
Sarcoid, CS psoriasiform sarcoid.

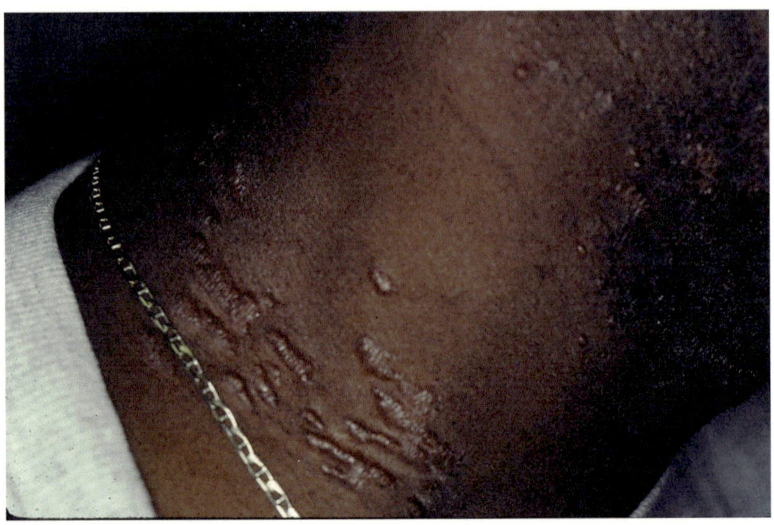

Figure 14.
Sarcoid, JS resembling pseudofolliculitis.

a minimal inflammatory infiltrate so called “naked” granulomas. Within these cells there can be foci of calcification: “Schaumann bodies” or intracytoplsmic stellate inclusions “asteroid bodies”. The granulomas are often through the dermis, but in some variants can involve the subcutis and have clinical features of a panniculitis (Darier-Roussy variant) (**Figure 25**) [21]. In contrast to infectious granulomas, there is usually no significant necrosis and at most mild fibrinoid change. With time the lesions may show hyalinization and fibrosis.

As many other conditions can show granulomatous histology, it is important that the pathologist is able to formulate a good clinicopathologic correlation. As sarcoid

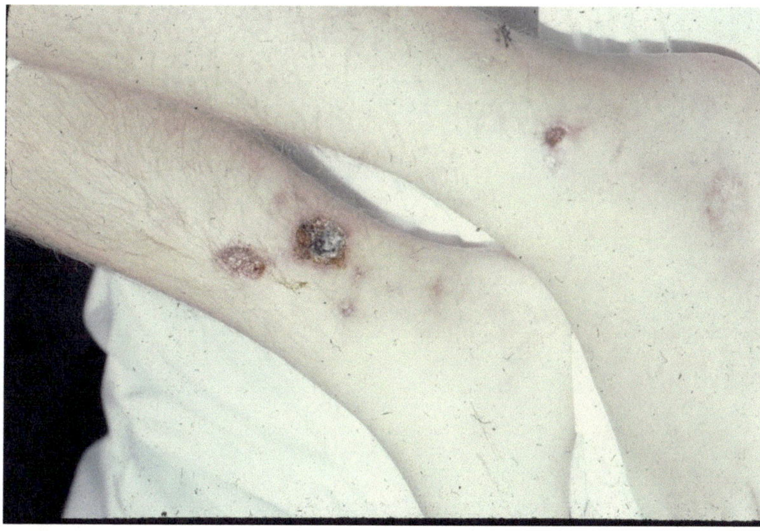

Figure 15.
Sarcoid, L stasis dermatitis-like.

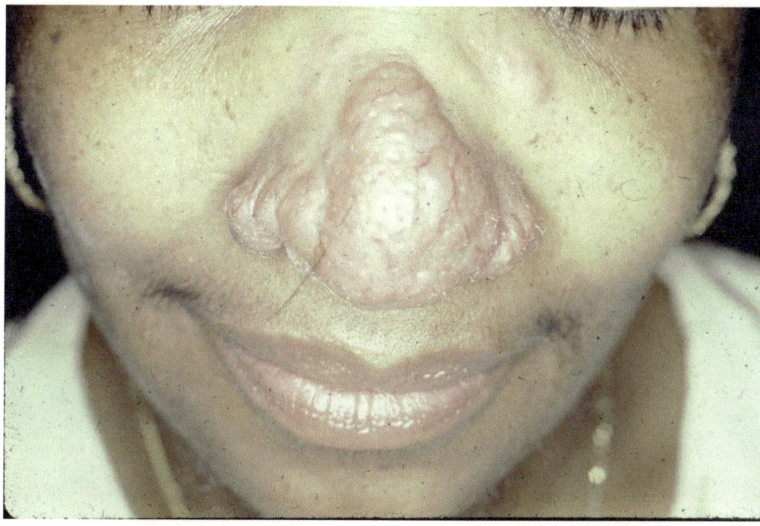

Figure 16.
Sarcoid, enlargement of nose resembling rhinophyma.

clinically can mimic other conditions, exacting criteria must be used to define the condition, as well as knowing the limitations of pathology. This is particularly true in dermatology and dermatopathology as many simulators exist.

The following disorders can mimic sarcoid: rosacea-like dermatoses, tuberculous leprosy, reactions to environmental injury (tattoos, metal and industrial exposures, foreign body reactions) lupus vulgaris, infectious granulomas, tuberculids, necrobiotic granulomas and granulomatous vasculitides.

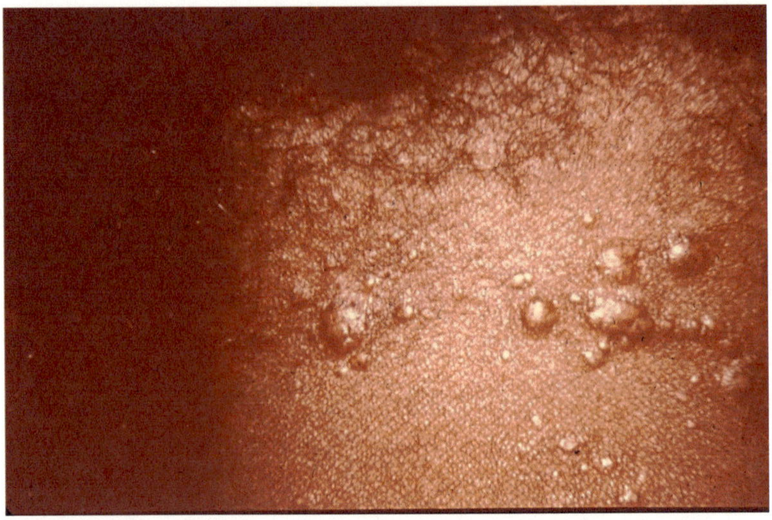

Figure 17.
Sarcoidosis, resembling acne nuchae keloidalis.

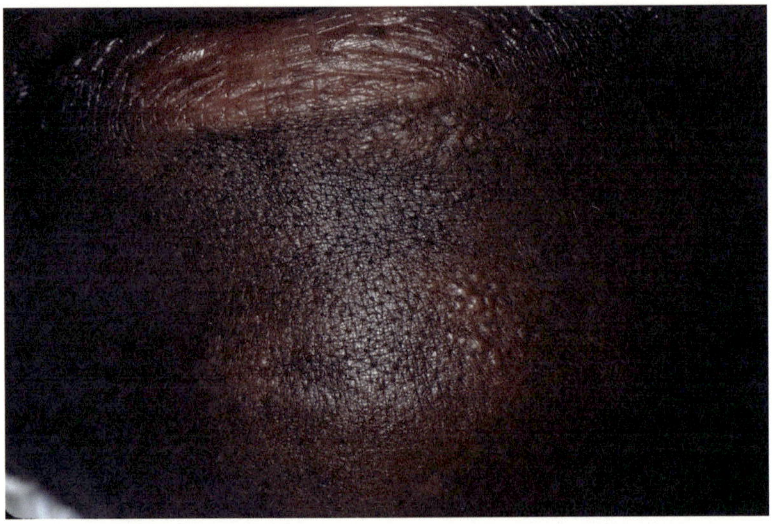

Figure 18.
Clusters of brown papules resembling lichen nitidus.

Granulomatous rosacea is an acneiform dermatosis, that can mimic sarcoid clinically and pathologically [22]. Certain clinical variants of the conditions, such perioral dermatitis, lupus miliaris disseminates faciei also occur commonly on facial skin – areas where sarcoid presents. If a granlulomatous condition is evident on facial skin, the pathologist must exercise care in defining it as sarcoid or not. In most types of granulomatous rosacea, there are histologic features which deviate from the typical presentation of sarcoid. First, the granulomatous are most often inflammatory, i.e., surrounded by mononuclear cells, particularly plasma cells. Second, in adjacent skin, there often are features of other types of rosacea – with other pustules

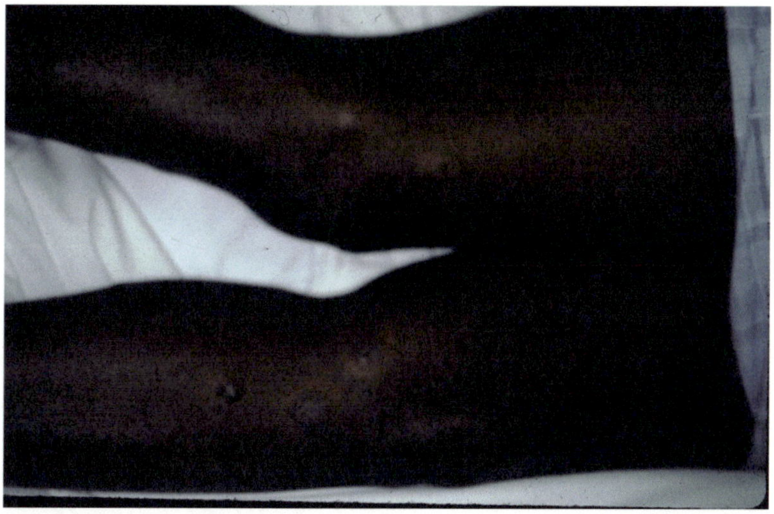

Figure 19.
Sarcoid, JW scars.

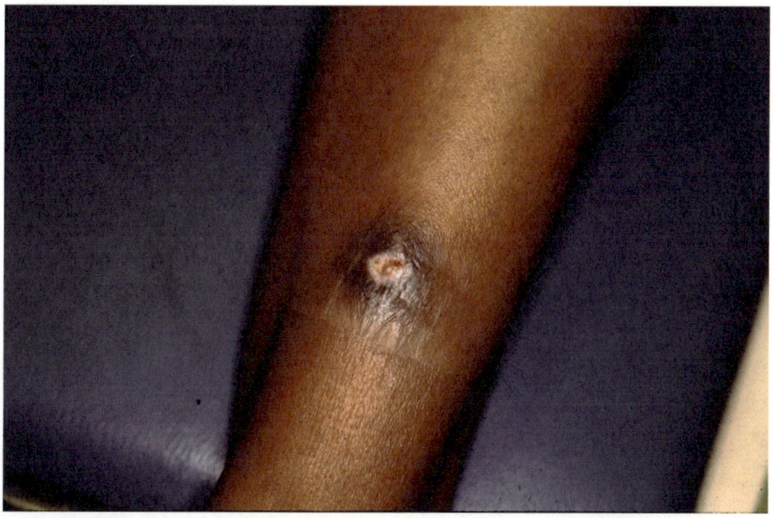

Figure 20.
Sarcoid, ulcerated scarlike.

or telangiectasia of the erythematotelangiectatic type (**Figure 26**). Despite these clues, there are rosacea like dermatoses, particularly childhood types – disseminated periorificial dermatitis, where these clues may not be present. In those cases, the pathologist should state their uncertainty in the report and advise that the diagnosis may have to be confirmed by other means – laboratory studies or clinical trials.

Tuberculoid leprosy may mimic sarcoid clinically with annular lesions but often there are other features that allow for a clinical distinction, such enlarged peripheral nerves, loss of sensation, anhidrosis or travel history. Pathologically, it can much more difficult. There can be nodular collections of epithelioid cells with a sparse infiltrate.

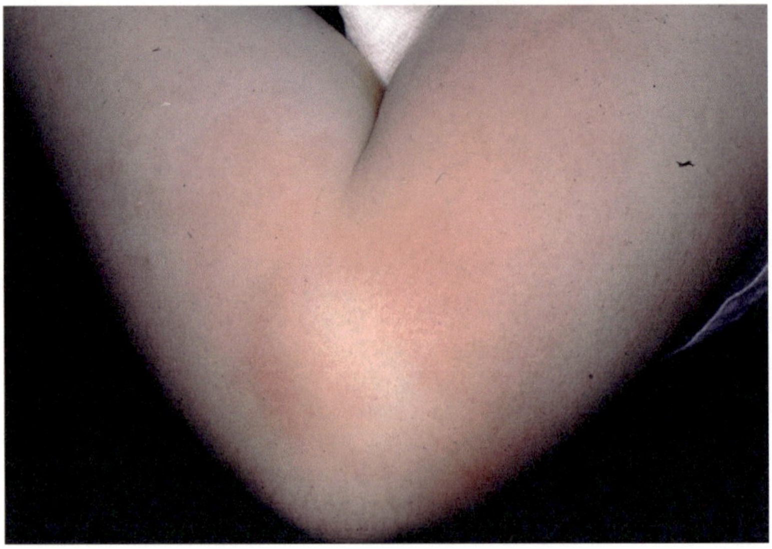

Figure 21.
Erythema Nodosum sarcoid.

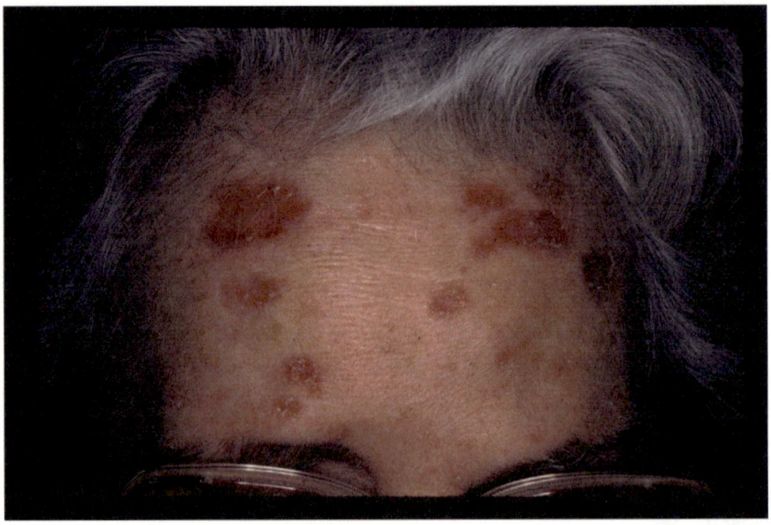

Figure 22.
Annular sarcoid.

Things to look for which favor tuberculoid leprosy: oval granulomas, following peripheral nerves and destruction of those nerves by the granulomas. Fite or auramine O stain can helpful for demonstrating organisms but more often than not the number of bacilli are few or undetectable.

Reactions to foreign substances can also mimic sarcoid. Reactions to tattoos may show sarcoidal, granulomas (**Figure 27**), corals, sea urchins, and cacti can show granulomatous histology. Sometimes the reaction can be of a foreign body type, and later become more sarcoidal [23]. Similar reactions may occur to heavy metals

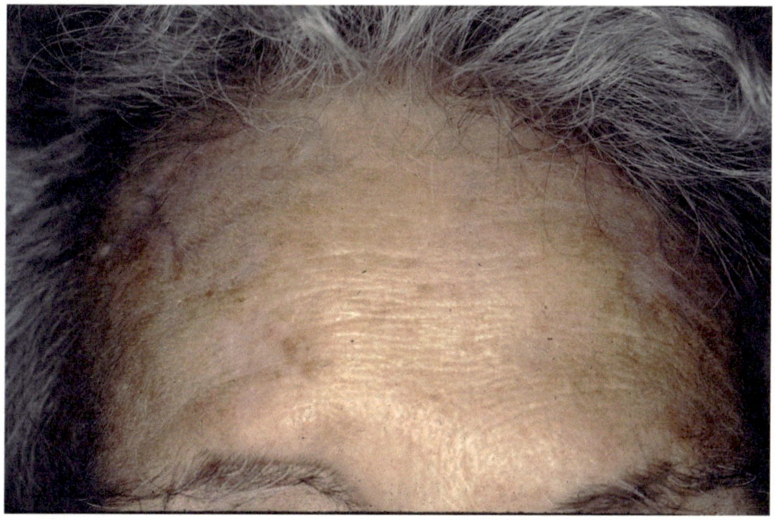

Figure 23.
Sarcoid, post Rx.

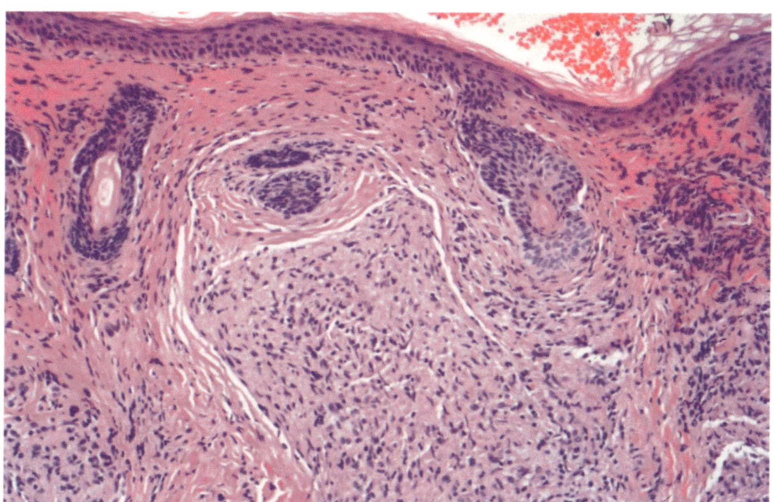

Figure 24.
Cutaneous sarcoid, histopathology H and E,10x.

(zicornium, beryllium). Even though these agents can cause this type of reaction, it still may be necessary to exclude sarcoidosis. Sarcoid can often localize to areas of antecedent injury –so called locus minoris resistentiae. Often it is necessary to state that localization of sarcoid cannot be excluded.

Infectious granulomas are also in the differential. This is perhaps the most important category to exclude unequivocally, as the therapy is the opposite of sarcoid – antimicrobial versus immunosuppressive. Principal among these are mycobacterial infections both atypical types and tuberculous. In general infectious mycobacterial reactions have some clue to their genesis – necrosis within the granulomas,

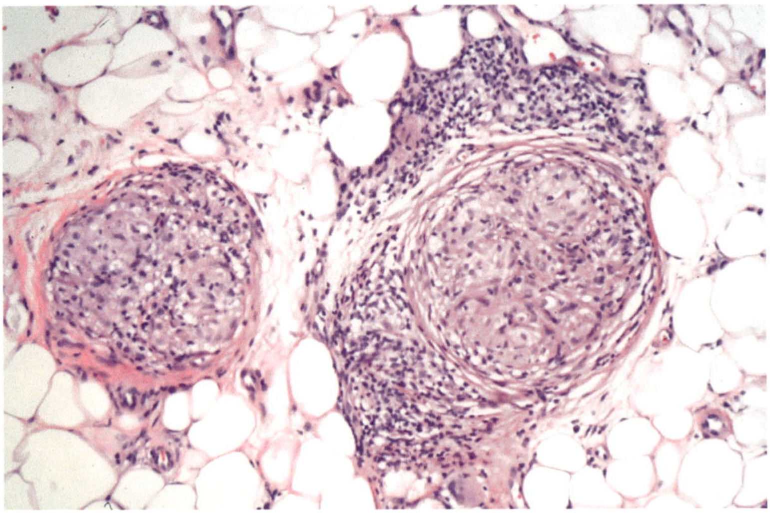

Figure 25.
Subcutaneous sarcoid, histopathology H and E, 10x.

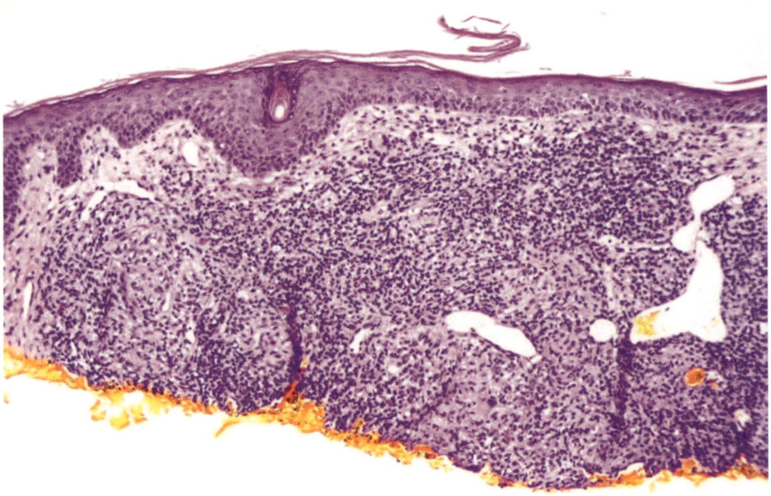

Figure 26.
Granulomatous rosacea, histopathology H and E, 10x.

an adjacent suppurative or mononuclear infiltrate, or epidermal hyperplasia. Unfortunately, particularly in rare subtypes of atypical mycobacteria, the distinction may be very difficult if not impossible. In those cases, sometimes the clinical parameters are paramount – do the lesions show sporotrichoid spread? Is there a recent onset? Is there a history of an occupational, or local exposure? In those equivocal cases, special stains, culture or PCR should be performed.

Other infections conditions can also show granulomas – deep fungal infections, and leishmania. Fortunately, organisms are usually easily visualized in the

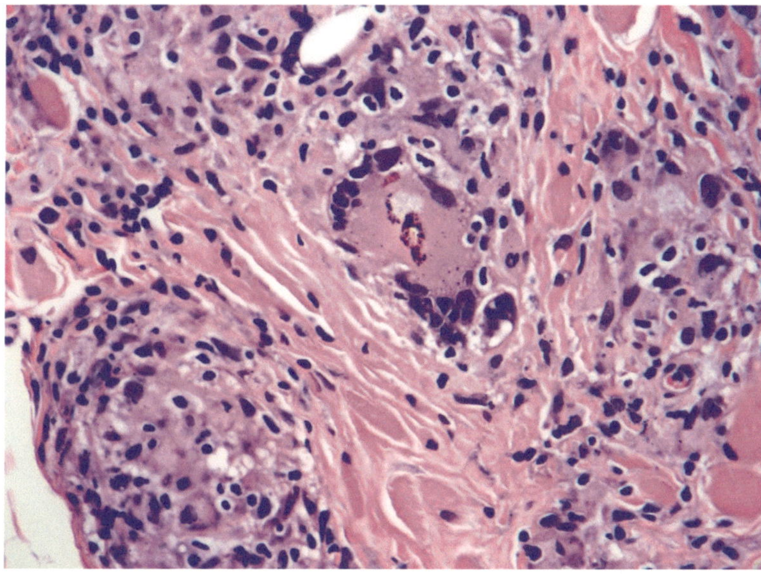

Figure 27.
Granulomatous reaction to tattoo, histopathology H and E, 20x.

acute and subacute stages, though with chronicity can be less evident. In addition to special stains, additional microbiologic studies may be needed to confirm the diagnosis.

Tuberculids refer to lesions that arise in patients as a hypersensitivity reaction to the tubercle bacilli, distant from the site of the primary infection. There are many clinical types – papulonecrotic tuberculids, lichen scrofulosorum, and erythema induratum [24]. These entities all show well defined granulomas often with necrosis but with limited evidence of an active infection. Treatment of the primary infection usually results in resolution of the process.

Other miscellaneous conditions can show granulomas. Metastatic Crohn's disease can show small granulomas distant from primary lesions of the disease [25]. Melkersson-Rosenthal syndrome and granulomatous cheilitis can also show small collections of epithelioid cells, often with adjacent lymphangiectasia [26]. Deep folliculitides, such as hidradenitis suppurativa, though often showing foreign body granulomas, can sometimes have a sarcoidal pathology as well. Certain necobiotic granuomas such as granuloma annulare can show sarcoid; lymphoproliferative disorders can show a focal granulatous histology [27]. In all of these conditions, the clinical appearance is paramount in making the correct diagnosis.

From this perspective the pathologic differential diagnosis of sarcoidosis is vast. Many other conditions can mimic and often the diagnosis is one of exclusion. In all cases it is essential the pathologist have access to clinical information and often clinical photographs; and that all special stains be performed as necessary: including infectious disease stains, acid fast, fite and other bacterial stains; other stains be performed if the differential includes a necrobiotic granuloma, such as shiktata, Voerhoeff von gieson and colloidal iron. If the granulomas are void of an inflammatory infiltrate, if there is no significant ulceration or substantial epidermal hyperplasia, the diagnosis can be suggested.

5. Summary

Sarcoid can be very variable in its clinical presentations and course. The systemic manifestations of sarcoid can mimic those of many conditions. Likewise, the cutaneous manifestations of sarcoid can be very variable and can mimic many cutaneous disorders. Clinicians must maintain a healthy level of suspicion when a diagnosis of sarcoid is considered.

Author details

Lily Lebwohl and Robert G. Phelps*
Departments of Dermatology and Pathology, Icahn School of Medicine at Mount Sinai, New York, New York, USA

*Address all correspondence to: rpdermpath@aol.com

References

[1] Spagnolo P, Rossi G, Trisolini R, Sverzellati N, Baughman RP, Wells AU. Pulmonary sarcoidosis. The Lancet Respiratory Medicine. 2018;**6**(5):389-402. DOI: 10.1016/S2213-2600(18)30064-X

[2] Markatis E, Afthinos A, Antonakis E, Papanikolaou IC. Cardiac sarcoidosis: diagnosis and management. Reviews in Cardiovascular Medicine. 2020;**21**(3):321-338. DOI: 10.31083/j.rcm.2020.03.102

[3] Calatroni M, Moroni G, Reggiani F, Ponticelli C. Renal sarcoidosis. Journal of Nephrology. 2023;**36**(1):5-15. DOI: 10.1007/s40620-022-01369-y

[4] Mañá J, Marcoval J, Graells J, Salazar A, Peyrí J, Pujol R. Cutaneous involvement in sarcoidosis. Relationship to systemic disease. Archives of Dermatology. 1997;**133**(7):882-888. DOI: 10.1001/archderm.1997.03890430098013

[5] Kundakci N, Erdem C. Leprosy: A great imitator. Clinics in Dermatology. 2019;**37**(3):200-212. DOI: 10.1016/j.clindermatol.2019.01.002

[6] Gurel MS, Tekin B, Uzun S. Cutaneous leishmaniasis: A great imitator. Clinics in Dermatology. 2020;**38**(2):140-151. DOI: 10.1016/j.clindermatol.2019.10.008

[7] Judson MA. Granulomatous Sarcoidosis Mimics. Frontiers in Medicine. 2021;**8**:680989. DOI: 10.3389/fmed.2021.680989

[8] Torralba KD, Quismorio FP Jr. Sarcoidosis and the rheumatologist. Current Opinion in Rheumatology. 2009;**21**(1):62-70. DOI: 10.1097/bor.0b013e32831dde88

[9] Shanks AM, Alluri R, Herriot R, Dempsey O. Misdiagnosis of common variable immune deficiency. BML Case Reports. 2014;**2014**:bcr2013202806. DOI: 10.1136/bcr-2013-202806

[10] Sarmento Tatagiba L, Bridi Pivatto L, Faccini-Martínez ÁA, Mendes Peçanha P, Grão Velloso TR, Santos Gonçalves S, et al. A case of paracoccidioidomycosis due to *Paracoccidioides lutzii* presenting sarcoid-like form. Medical Mycology Case Reports. 2017;**19**:6-8. DOI: 10.1016/j.mmcr.2017.09.002

[11] Alexandra G, Claudia G. Lymphomatoid granulomatosis mimicking cancer and sarcoidosis. Annals of Hematology. 2019;**98**(5):1309-1311. DOI: 10.1007/s00277-018-3505-4

[12] Ezeh N, Caplan A, Rosenbach M, Imadojemu S. Cutaneous Sarcoidosis. Dermatologic Clinics. 2023;**41**(3):455-470. DOI: 10.1016/j.det.2023.02.012

[13] Amschler K, Seitz CS. Kutane Manifestationen bei Sarkoidose [cutaneous manifestations of sarcoidosis]. Zeitschrift für Rheumatologie. 2017;**76**(5):382-390. German. DOI: 10.1007/s00393-017-0290-8

[14] Bargagli E, Prasse A. Sarcoidosis: A review for the internist. Internal and Emergency Medicine. 2018;**13**(3):325-331. DOI: 10.1007/s11739-017-1778-6

[15] Arkema EV, Cozier YC. Sarcoidosis epidemiology: Recent estimates of incidence, prevalence and risk factors. Current Opinion in Pulmonary Medicine. 2020;**26**(5):527-534. DOI: 10.1097/MCP.0000000000000715

[16] Spagnolo P, Maier LA. Genetics in sarcoidosis. Current Opinion in

Pulmonary Medicine. 2021;**27**(5):423-429. DOI: 10.1097/MCP.0000000000000798

[17] Wills AB, Adjemian J, Fontana JR, et al. Sarcoidosis-associated hospitalizations in the United States, 2002 to 2012. Annals of the American Thoracic Society. 2018;**15**(12):1490-1493

[18] Hena KM. Sarcoidosis epidemiology: Race matters. Frontiers in Immunology. 2020;**11**:537382. DOI: 10.3389/fimmu.2020.537382

[19] Neville E, Walker AN, James DG. Prognostic factors predicting the outcome of sarcoidosis: An analysis of 818 patients. The Quarterly Journal of Medicine. 1983;**52**(208):525-533

[20] Dai C, Shih S, Ansari A, Kwak Y, Sami N. Biologic therapy in the treatment of cutaneous sarcoidosis: A literature review. American Journal of Clinical Dermatology. 2019;**20**(3):409-422. DOI: 10.1007/s40257-019-00428-8

[21] Marcoval J et al. Histopathological features of subcutaneous sarcoidosis. The American Journal of Dermatopathology. 2020;**42**(4):233-243

[22] Lee GL et al. Granulomatous rosacea and periorificial dermatitis: Controversies and review of management and treatment. Dermatologic Clinics. 2015;**33**(3):447-455

[23] Lim D et al. Sarcoidal reaction in a tattoo. The New England Journal of Medicine. 2020;**382**(8):744

[24] Feuer J, Phelps RG, Kerr LD. Erythema nodosum vs erythema induratum: A crucial distinction enabling recognition of occult tuberculosis. Journal of Clinical Rheumatology. 1995;**1**:357-362

[25] Emanuel PO, Phelps RG. Metastatic Crohn's disease: A histopathologic study of 12 cases. Journal of Cutaneous Pathology. May 2008;**35**(5):457-461

[26] Lenskaya V, de Moll EH, Bhatt S, Hussein S, Phelps RG. The subtlety of granulomatous mycosis Fungoides: A retrospective case-series study and proposal of novel multimodal diagnostic approach and literature review. American Journal of Dermatopathology. 2022;**44**(8):559-567

[27] Lenskaya V, Panji P, de Moll EH, Christian K, Phelps RG. Oral lymphangiectasia and gastrointestinal Crohn disease. Journal of Cutaneous Pathology. 2020;**47**(11):1080-1084

Chapter 4

Ocular Manifestations of Sarcoidosis

Abhishek Sethi, Corrina P. Azarcon and Monique Munro

Abstract

Sarcoidosis is a complex granulomatous systemic inflammatory disease that can affect the eye and its adnexa. Ocular sarcoidosis is a leading cause of inflammatory eye disease that can result in significant visual impairment. Ocular inflammation can manifest with a wide range of clinical presentations and can involve almost any structure within or around the orbit causing uveitis, episcleritis/scleritis, eyelid anomalies, conjunctival granulomas, optic neuropathy, lacrimal gland enlargement, glaucoma, and/or cataract. The diagnosis of ocular sarcoidosis is typically established based on the presence of characteristic ophthalmologic findings, along with a positive tissue biopsy or bilateral hilar adenopathy on chest imaging. Topical, periocular, and systemic corticosteroids are commonly used to treat ocular sarcoidosis. Chronic cases or refractory cases may warrant immunomodulator therapy. Visual prognosis is contingent on severity of inflammation, time to treatment, and secondary ocular complications. This chapter will discuss the presentation, diagnosis, treatment, and prognosis of patients with ocular sarcoidosis.

Keywords: granulomatous uveitis, ocular granulomatosis, ocular sarcoidosis, sarcoid uveitis, sarcoidosis-related uveitis

1. Introduction

Ocular disease may be the first manifestation of systemic sarcoidosis [1]. The reported incidence of ocular involvement in sarcoidosis ranges from 13 to 79%, with approximately 20–30% presenting with ocular symptoms as the primary manifestation [1–4]. Ocular sarcoidosis can affect many ocular tissues simultaneously with several clinical presentations; thus, diagnosis can be challenging. Typical ocular symptoms include redness, decreased vision, photophobia, and/or eye pain.

The most common presentation of ocular sarcoidosis is uveitis [5]. Uveitis is a term used by ophthalmologists to describe inflammation of the uveal tissues, which includes the iris, ciliary body, and choroid. Uveitis can be classified by the anatomic location of the observed inflammation seen by the ophthalmologist using the slit lamp to examine the eye. The most universally accepted formal uveitis classification and grading scheme used by ophthalmologists was published by the Standardization of Uveitis Nomenclature (SUN) Working Group [1, 5]. The SUN Working Group is an international uveitis collaboration and has developed a classification criteria for the leading causes of ocular inflammation, which includes sarcoidosis-associated uveitis. When classifying by anatomic location, uveitis can present as anterior, intermediate, posterior, or panuveitis. The typical presentation of sarcoid uveitis is characterized by granulomatous inflammation with large mutton-fat keratic precipitates (KP), nodules on the pupillary margin (Koeppe nodules) or within the iris stroma (Busacca nodules), or choroidal granulomas (**Figure 1**) [6]. This chapter will describe these ocular findings, diagnosis, and treatment strategies. An overview of ocular manifestations of sarcoidosis is displayed in **Table 1**.

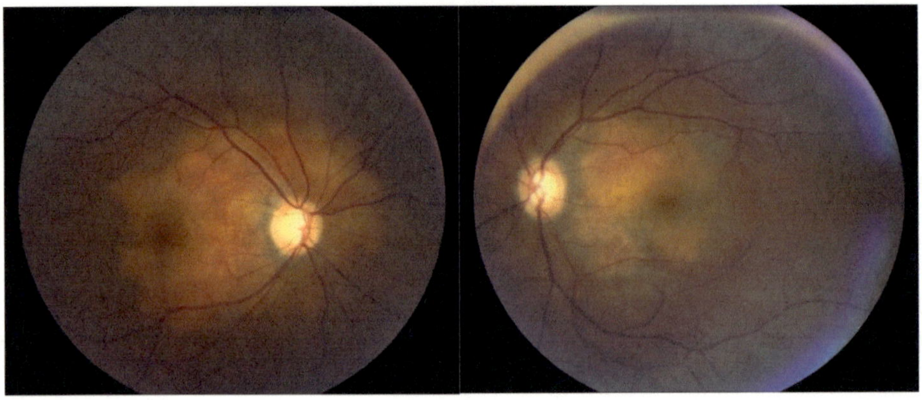

Figure 1.
Bilateral choroidal granulomas in a 33-year-old female with sarcoidosis (photo courtesy of Calgary retina consultants).

Ocular structures	Findings
Eyelids	Eyelid granuloma, madarosis (loss of eyelashes), poliosis (whitening of lashes), entropion, trichiasis, lagoghthalmos (if associated with facial palsy)
Extraocular muscles and orbital tissues	Strabismus, proptosis, optic nerve compression
Conjunctiva	Conjunctival nodules, conjunctivitis, symblepharon
Sclera and Episclera	Episcleritis, scleritis
Cornea	Keratoconjunctivitis sicca
Iris	Iris nodules, posterior synechiae
Anterior chamber	Inflammatory cell, KP
Trabecular meshwork	Angle granulomas, peripheral anterior synechiae
Lens	Cataract, posterior synechiae
Vitreous	Vitreous cell, snowballs, snowbanks
Retina and choroid	Retinitis, vasculitis, CME, Choroiditis, Choroidal granulomas
Optic nerve and visual pathways	Relative afferent pupillary defects, visual field defects, abnormal eye movement, optic nerve inflammation or granulomas

Table 1.
Ocular manifestations of sarcoidosis (adapted from Ref. [1]).

2. Demographics

Uveitis has been reported in 30–70% of ocular sarcoidosis cases and is one of the most common manifestations of the disease [1]. Among patients with systemic sarcoidosis, females are more likely to develop ocular involvement compared to males [1]. The age distribution of ocular sarcoidosis in adults demonstrates a bimodal presentation with peaks of incidence between the ages of 20–30 years and 50–60 years [1]. Sarcoidosis is less common in children and in one report accounted for approximately 1–3% of pediatric uveitis in ophthalmology referral centers in the United States [1]. Sarcoid uveitis typically involves both eyes, and approximately 90% are chronic. Thus, awareness of ocular manifestations is important for physicians who regularly see patients with sarcoidosis [1].

Individuals of pigmented race with biopsy-proven sarcoidosis have a higher likelihood of developing ocular involvement compared to Caucasians. There is also evidence for the allelic variations at the HLA-DRB1 locus as a contributing factor for sarcoidosis; specifically, the HLA-DRB1*0401 allele has been associated with ocular involvement [1]. Patients with ocular sarcoidosis appear to have less systemic involvement albeit with varying reported rates. For instance, out of 294 patients with sarcoid uveitis, only 2.4% of them developed cardiac involvement [7], while another study reported 4.4% of cardiac sarcoidosis in a retrospective cohort of sarcoid uveitis [8].

3. Ocular manifestations of sarcoidosis

3.1 Anterior segment findings

The anterior segment of the eye includes the cornea, anterior chamber, iris, and lens. Anterior chamber inflammation is the most common ocular presentation of sarcoidosis. In one study, anterior chamber involvement was detected in 42 out of 46 patients (91%) with biopsy-confirmed sarcoid uveitis. Thirty-eight of these patients had solely anterior chamber involvement [9]. Characteristic clinical presentations associated with anterior chamber inflammation include redness, eye pain, decreased vision, and photophobia. Pain associated with uveitis can occur secondary to ciliary muscle spasm or elevated intraocular pressure (IOP). Elevated IOP may be secondary to blockage of the aqueous outflow pathway, known as the trabecular meshwork, by inflammatory cells, sarcoid nodules, or adhesion of the peripheral iris to the peripheral cornea (peripheral anterior synechiae) [1, 6]. Keratic precipitates are visualized when anterior chamber leukocytes precipitate onto the posterior surface of the cornea [1, 6]. The size of these KPs varies, and larger KPs are typically seen in cases of granulomatous uveitis. Granulomatous uveitis is a specific pattern of uveitis that is seen with a small number of uveitis causes and includes sarcoidosis. Granulomatous uveitis must have at least one of the following clinical signs: large mutton-fat KP, iris or trabecular meshwork nodules, and/or choroidal granulomas. However, these clinical findings may not be observed in all cases of ocular sarcoidosis, especially in early or mild disease [1].

Iris involvement is also common. Untreated anterior uveitis can lead to iris adhesions to the anterior lens capsule (posterior synechiae) can cause an irregularly shaped pupil [1]. Severe posterior synechiae can lead to a completely occluded pupil known as iris bombe, and this is often associated with increased IOP. Cataract formation can develop secondary to persistent inflammation as well as treatment with topical corticosteroids [1, 6].

3.2 Posterior segment findings

The posterior segment of the eye includes the following eye structures: vitreous humor, the retina, the choroid, and the optic nerve. Posterior uveitis is less common than anterior uveitis but is often more vision threatening [6].

Intermediate uveitis mainly affects the vitreous and peripheral retina and is a common presentation of ocular sarcoidosis. Symptoms of intermediate uveitis include floaters and decreased vision. In contrast to patients with anterior segment inflammation, patients with intermediate uveitis tend to experience less pain. On examination with the slit lamp biomicroscope, vitreous cells may be observed. Cystoid macular edema (CME) can be seen on fundus examination or with the aid of imaging tools such as optical coherence tomography. Inflammatory cells can accumulate inferiorly in the vitreous cavity along the pars plana. When the inflammatory debris in this area collect in sheets, they are called "snowbanks"; meanwhile, when found in focal consolidations, they are known as "snowballs" or "string of pearls" [1, 6].

Inflammation of the retina and choroid, respectively known as retinitis and choroiditis, may also be seen in ocular sarcoidosis. Vascular inflammation can present as perivascular sheathing. Deposition of white-yellow perivascular exudates in the retina alongside the retinal veins and is called "candle-wax drippings" [1, 6]. Generally, ocular sarcoidosis does not cause retinal vascular occlusion but has been reported in approximately 5% of cases [5, 6]. If occlusion occurs acutely or with chronic or untreated retinal vasculitis or intermediate uveitis, retinal neovascularization may develop. This can cause vitreous hemorrhage if severe. Fluorescein angiography is an imaging modality that can assess the retinal vasculature and severity of retinal inflammation. Posterior uveitis is generally associated with more frequent relapses and a poorer visual prognosis [6].

Similar to sarcoid granulomas observed in the other parts of the body, granulomas can develop in the retina and choroid. These granulomas may be unifocal or multifocal and can vary in size. Visual changes can vary depending on the location of these granulomas and can range to asymptomatic if located in the peripheral retina to severe vision decline if located in the macula, the retinal area responsible for central vision. Exudative retinal detachments can be associated with larger granulomas, although this finding is rare [1, 5, 6].

Optic nerve findings in sarcoidosis may include optic nerve granulomas, optic disc edema, or disc hyperemia. If inflammation is severe or chronic, optic atrophy with irreversibly impaired vision may result. Pupillary abnormalities, such as a relative pupillary defect can be noted on exam with optic nerve involvement or damage [1].

Finally, panuveitis describes inflammation affecting all structures of the uvea and accounts for approximately 37% of sarcoid uveitis by the SUN working group [5]. Sarcoidosis is the most frequently systemic disease associated with panuveitis [6].

3.3 Orbital involvement

The orbit includes the lacrimal gland, orbital fat, extraocular muscles, and the optic nerve sheath [1]. Infiltration or inflammation of the lacrimal gland and muscles from ocular sarcoidosis may present with a palpable eyelid mass and eyelid swelling [1]. Other symptoms indicating orbital involvement include globe displacement, ptosis, proptosis, pain, redness and tearing. Double vision (diplopia) can occur if cranial nerves are compressed or by mass effect. Vision loss can result in severe cases if the optic nerve is compressed.

Coexisting systemic sarcoidosis are present in approximately 34–50% of biopsy-proven orbital sarcoidosis [1]. Orbital sarcoidosis lesions tend to be well circumscribed on imaging in 85–90% of patients, with 10–15% of diffuse or infiltrative patterns noted [1]. On histopathology and gross examination, orbital lesions tend to be solid as opposed to cystic [10].

The lacrimal gland is the most common orbital structure affected by sarcoidosis [1]. Patients with lacrimal gland involvement may or may not be symptomatic. The lacrimal gland produces the aqueous component of the tear film; therefore, patients may complain of dry eye symptoms when the gland is infiltrated by sarcoid granulomas or is inflamed. If the lacrimal gland is significantly enlarged, symptoms secondary to mass effect can result as mentioned above.

3.4 Eyelid and ocular surface

Eyelid granulomas may vary in size from small papules to larger lesions that can distort eyelid architecture [1]. Madarosis or loss of eyelashes may occur but is typically seen with more invasive and destructive eyelid tumors. Infiltration or inflammation of the lacrimal drainage system, which consists of the canaliculi, nasolacrimal sac, and nasolacrimal duct, may manifest as excessive tearing [1].

Corneal involvement can manifest as superficial punctate keratitis secondary to dry eye syndrome, known as keratoconjunctivitis sicca. This occurs secondary to lacrimal gland inflammation/infiltration. Episcleritis and scleritis are uncommonly associated with sarcoidosis [1]. Scleritis may present as anterior diffuse, anterior nodular, or posterior scleritis. Common symptoms of scleritis include ocular pain and redness. Vision is often unaffected [1].

Conjunctival involvement is common, and nodules have been reported in 40% of cases [2]. However, granulomas in this area tend to be small and asymptomatic. Conjunctivitis can be mild with ocular redness and follicular conjunctivitis or can be severe with scarring, symblepharon and fornix shortening. Larger granulomas can mimic conjunctival tumors [1]. Conjunctival granulomas may present as white-yellow, discrete infiltrates and can vary in size. Sarcoid conjunctival nodules are commonly observed at the palpebral conjunctivae; however, they may also be located at other locations [1].

3.5 Glaucoma

Elevated IOP can be seen secondary to anterior chamber sarcoid uveitis. As discussed above, anterior chamber inflammation can cause iris adhesions to the trabecular meshwork (peripheral anterior synechiae) resulting in angle closure glaucoma and elevated IOP [1]. These patients can be managed with ocular hypotensive eye drops but may ultimately require glaucoma surgery. Elevated IOP can also be caused by orbital mass effect and prolonged steroid therapy. The latter is thought to be secondary to changes in the microstructure of trabecular meshwork, resulting in swelling and an increase in outflow resistance of aqueous fluid [11].

3.6 Neurosarcoidosis

Visual symptoms of neurosarcoidosis are associated with the location of granuloma formation and inflammation. Symptoms include decreased vision and visual field defects, papilledema secondary to increased intracranial pressure, abnormal eye movement, pupillary abnormalities, and peripheral neuropathy [1]. Cranial neuropathy involving the optic and facial nerves can occur secondary to neurosarcoidosis. As a result, facial paresis is a common presentation due to parotid gland inflammation. Additionally, lower motor neuron facial paresis can cause ipsilateral poor eyelid closure, which can result in exposure keratopathy and possible corneal ulcers [1].

4. Diagnosis

Sarcoidosis is a difficult diagnosis for clinicians given that it can involve many organs, ocular tissues, and may manifest in different clinical presentations. This condition most commonly affects the lungs and hilar lymph nodes [1, 5]. However, many patients are asymptomatic and may be diagnosed upon routine exam, further complicating initiation of timely treatment. The diagnosis of sarcoidosis includes three important criteria: (1) consistent clinical presentation, (2) presence of non-caseating granulomas in one or more tissue samples, and (3) exclusion of other causes of granulomatous disorders [6]. The World Association of Sarcoidosis and Other Granulomatous Disorders (WASOG) created consensus criteria to categorize the likelihood of a sarcoid diagnosis that has been revised and updated over time. For example, sarcoidosis was highly probable given symptoms of uveitis or findings of bilateral hilar lymph nodes, or perilymphatic nodules on chest computed tomography scan (CT). It was considered probable with cranial nerve infiltration, lacrimal gland swelling, and/or upper lobe or diffuse infiltrates on chest CT. Arthralgia and/or localized infiltrates on chest CT suggested a possible but less likely diagnosis [6]. It is also important to rule out differential diagnoses of ocular sarcoidosis which include infections such as tuberculosis and malignancies such as lymphoma [6]. The Classification Criteria for Sarcoid Uveitis published by the SUN Working Group is shown in **Table 2**.

Generally, sarcoidosis should be high on the differential in cases where there are multiple ocular tissues involved. Ophthalmologists will initiate a focused uveitis workup depending on the pattern of inflammation and ocular findings observed. The gold standard for diagnosis of sarcoidosis includes tissue biopsy from an affected area from the lungs, lymph nodes, skin, conjunctiva, lacrimal glands, or orbital tissues [1]. However, given that a biopsy is not feasible in many cases, guidelines from the International Workshop on Ocular Sarcoidosis have been published which recommend laboratory tests when a biopsy is not performed or results negative [12]. Imaging, such as a chest x-ray or chest CT can help confirm diagnosis when sarcoidosis is suspected. Patients may also have elevated biomarkers including calcium, angiotensin converting enzyme (ACE), and/or lysozyme [1].

5. Treatment

Generally, sarcoid uveitis is treated with corticosteroids. The selection of the steroid administration route (e.g. periocular, intraocular, systemic) and the addition of corticosteroid-sparing immunomodulators is primarily determined by the extent

Criteria
1. Compatible uveitic picture, either
a. Anterior uveitis OR
b. Intermediate or anterior/intermediate uveitis OR
c. Posterior uveitis with either choroiditis (paucifocal choroidal nodule(s) or multifocal choroiditis) OR
d. Panuveitis with choroiditis or retinal vascular sheathing or retinal vascular occlusion
AND 2. Evidence of sarcoidosis, either
a. Tissue biopsy demonstrating non-caseating granulomata OR
b. Bilateral hilar adenopathy on chest imaging
Exclusions
1. Positive serology for syphilis using a treponemal test 2. Evidence of infection with Mycobacterium tuberculosis,* either
a. Histologically- or microbiologically-confirmed infection with M. tuberculosis† OR
b. Positive interferon-γ release assay (IGRA)‡ OR
c. Positive tuberculin skin test§

**Routine exclusion of tuberculosis is not required in areas where tuberculosis is non-endemic but should be performed in areas where tuberculosis is endemic or in tuberculosis-exposed patients. With evidence of latent tuberculosis in a patient with a uveitic syndrome compatible with either sarcoidosis or tubercular uveitis and bilateral hilar adenopathy, the classification as sarcoid uveitis can be made only with biopsy confirmation of sarcoidosis (and therefore exclusion of tuberculosis).*
†E.g. Biopsy, fluorochrome stain, culture, or polymerase chain reaction based assay.
‡E.g. Quantiferon-gold or T-spot.
§E.g. Purified protein derivative (PPD) skin test; a positive result should be >10 mm induration.

Table 2.
Classification criteria for sarcoid uveitis (adapted from the SUN working Group[5]).

of inflammation, ocular or adnexal tissues involved, and whether the inflammation is unilateral or bilateral. Furthermore, the use of topical cycloplegic eye drops can help relieve pain from ciliary spasm and to reduce posterior synechiae [1]. For scleritis, non-steroidal anti-inflammatory drugs (NSAIDs) are usually prescribed as first-line therapy. In uveitis with posterior segment involvement, regional corticosteroid injections such as triamcinolone acetonide (1–4 mg) and steroid implants can be considered. Tumor necrosis factor (TNF)-alpha inhibitors, namely, infliximab, adalimumab, etanercept, and golimumab, are considered as novel treatment options, although scientific evidence remains limited to small studies [1].

Common ocular complications of ocular sarcoidosis include cataract, epiretinal membrane formation and glaucoma, and patients need to be regularly assessed for the development of these conditions [1]. Corticosteroid therapy should be managed carefully in patients with elevated IOP. Systemic immunosuppressant medications also need to be monitored for systemic side effects.

6. Prognosis

The visual prognosis of ocular sarcoidosis is highly dependent on the severity of inflammation, chronicity of underlying disease, time to presentation to an ophthalmologist, and presence of ocular complications [1]. One paper which followed sarcoid uveitis patients over a median of 4 years determined that 54% of patients retained normal vision acuity (20/40 or better), and only 4.6% of patients lost vision to worse than 20/120 bilaterally [13]. Generally, regular follow-up and medication compliance are essential for a favorable prognosis.

7. Conclusion

A multidisciplinary approach is essential to optimize treatment outcomes for both ocular and systemic manifestations of sarcoidosis. Effective communication and collaboration between ophthalmologists and non-ophthalmologists are key to providing comprehensive care. With early diagnosis and appropriate management, visual prognosis for patients with ocular sarcoidosis is generally good. Larger longitudinal prospective studies are recommended to continue to advance the guidelines on management of patients with sarcoid uveitis.

Acknowledgements

The authors acknowledge Calgary Retina Consultants for providing clinical photos.

Conflict of interest

The authors declare no conflict of interest.

Author details

Abhishek Sethi[1], Corrina P. Azarcon[2] and Monique Munro[2]*

1 University of Illinois at Chicago, College of Medicine, Chicago, IL, United States

2 Department of Surgery, Section of Ophthalmology, University of Calgary, Calgary, Alberta, Canada

*Address all correspondence to: moniquepmunro@gmail.com

References

[1] Pasadhika S, Rosenbaum JT. Ocular sarcoidosis. Clinics in Chest Medicine. 2015;**36**:669-683. DOI: 10.1016/j.ccm.2015.08.009

[2] Rothova A. Ocular involvement in sarcoidosis. The British Journal of Ophthalmology. 2000;**84**:110-116. DOI: 10.1136/bjo.84.1.110

[3] Atmaca LS, Atmaca-Sönmez P, Idil A, KumbasarÖÖ,ÇelikG.Ocularinvolvement in sarcoidosis. Ocular Immunology and Inflammation. 2009;**17**:91-94. DOI: 10.1080/09273940802596526

[4] Heiligenhaus A, Wefelmeyer D, Wefelmeyer E, Rösel M, Schrenk M. The eye as a common site for the early clinical manifestation of sarcoidosis. Ophthalmic Research. 2011;**46**:9-12. DOI: 10.1159/000321947

[5] Standardization of Uveitis Nomenclature (SUN) Working Group. Classification criteria for sarcoidosis-associated uveitis. American Journal of Ophthalmology. 2021;**228**:220-230. DOI: 10.1016/j.ajo.2021.03.047

[6] Giorguitti S, Jacquot R, El Jammal T, Bert A, Jamilloux Y, Kodjikian L, et al. Sarcoidosis-related uveitis: A review. Journal of Clinical Medicine. 2023;**12**(9):3194. DOI: 10.3390/jcm12093194

[7] Richard M, Jamilloux Y, Courand P-Y, et al. Cardiac sarcoidosis is uncommon in patients with isolated sarcoid uveitis: Outcome of 294 cases. Journal of Clinical Medicine. 2021;**10**(10):2146. DOI: 10.3390/jcm10102146

[8] Niederer RL, Ma SP, Wilsher ML, et al. Systemic associations of sarcoid uveitis: Correlation with uveitis phenotype and ethnicity. American Journal of Ophthalmology. 2021;**229**:169-175. DOI: 10.1016/j.ajo.2021.03.003

[9] Crick RP, Hoyle C, Smellie H. The eyes in sarcoidosis. The British Journal of Ophthalmology. 1961;**45**(7):461-481. DOI: 10.1136/bjo.45.7.461

[10] Demirci H, Christianson MD. Orbital and adnexal involvement in sarcoidosis: Analysis of clinical features and systemic disease In 30 cases. American Journal of Ophthalmology. 2010;**151**(6):1074-1080. DOI: 10.1016/j.ajo.2010.12.011

[11] Phulke S, Kaushik S, Kaur S, et al. Steroid-induced glaucoma: An avoidable irreversible blindness. Journal of Current Glaucoma Practice. 2017;**11**(2):67-72. DOI: 10.5005/jp-journals-l0028-1226

[12] Herbort CP, Rao NA, Mochizuki M. International criteria for the diagnosis of ocular sarcoidosis: Results of the first international workshop on ocular sarcoidosis (IWOS). Ocular Immunology and Inflammation. 2009;**17**(3):160-169. DOI: 10.1080/09273940902818861

[13] Edelsten C, Pearson A, Joynes E, Stanford MR, Graham EM. The ocular and systemic prognosis of patients presenting with sarcoid uveitis. Eye. 1999;**13**:748-753. DOI: 10.1038/eye.1999.221

Chapter 5

Renal Sarcoidosis: One Disease, Different Kidney Involvements

Francesco Rastelli, Luisa Benozzi and Stefano Cusinato

Abstract

Renal sarcoidosis has a low frequency, from 0.1% to 0.2%, considering American monocentric cohorts of about 10,000 native kidney biopsies performed in 10-year period. Acute kidney injury (AKI), occurring in <1% of patients, brings sarcoidosis to nephrologist's attention. AKI in sarcoidosis is mainly due to hypercalcemia and sarcoid granulomatous interstitial nephritis (sGIN), the hallmark pathological finding of the disease. AKI related to hypercalcemia generally responds to steroids. At the contrary, not always all sGIN-AKI has a benign prognosis. This chapter will describe the widest casistics of renal sarcoidosis, considering the predictive value of clinical features, laboratory, radiological parameters, and histological patterns regarding induction therapy response to AKI. Rarely sarcoidosis is life-threatening: fatal events could occur during AKI or during the progression from chronic kidney disease (CKD) to end-stage renal disease (ESRD), a high-risk condition for cardiovascular, infectious, and oncological events. AKI to CKD transition due to specific injury of renal sarcoidosis is one of the most interesting aspects for nephrologists, as the reason why only a minority of sGIN cases will develop AKI: generally, sGIN is s a silent finding observed at autopsy in 7–23% of sarcoidosis patients.

Keywords: renal sarcoidosis, sarcoid granulomatous interstitial nephritis (sGIN), renal granulomas, acute kidney injury (AKI), renal failure, chronic kidney disease (CKD), hypercalcemia, hypercalciuria, sarcoidosis-associated renal involvements (SARI), sarcoidosis-associated hypercalciuria, nephrocalcinosis, vitamin D, 25-dihydroxyvitamin D, 1,25-dihydroxyvitamin D, parathyroid hormone-related peptide, giant cells, steroids, interstitial infiltrate, interstitial fibrosis, renal sarcoidosis phenotypes

1. Introduction

Sarcoidosis (S) is an idiopathic multisystemic granulomatous disorder, histologically characterized by epithelioid noncaseating granulomas which involve primarily lungs, mediastinum, lymph nodes, liver, eyes, and skin. All organs could be affected by the disease that rarely strikes kidneys, central nervous system, and heart [1]. In susceptible hosts, an abnormal T-helper 1 response to an unknown, not degradable antigen stimulates macrophages and dendritic cells to transform into epithelioid cells and to fuse together into multinucleate giant cells. In 1933 for the first time, Garland and Thomson described noncaseating sarcoid granulomas in the kidney [2].

The nodular inflammatory infiltrate in the renal interstitium characterizing sarcoid granulomatous interstitial nephritis (sGIN) includes one or more distinct aggregates of epithelioid cells as large as a glomerulus with or without multinucleate giant cells and lymphocytes in outer layers [3].

2. Renal sarcoidosis definition

sGIN is the classic pathological lesion of renal S, but there are many other forms of renal involvement. We can distinguish sarcoidosis-associated renal involvements (SARI) from renal sarcoidosis (RS): SARI is any renal manifestation of S, even functional as hypercalciuria and hypercalcemia. The term RS entails compatible renal histopathology. The spectrum of SARI can be divided into two groups, according to the presence of renal failure (**Table 1**). The same SARI may occur with or without renal failure, as observed in hypercalcemia and sGIN.

3. Disturbances of calcium and vitamin D

3.1 Frequency of hypercalciuria

Hypercalciuria (defined as urinary calcium >300 mg/day) is the more common SARI. It results from both an increased glomerular calcium filtration and a decreased calcium tubular reabsorption due to a PTH suppression caused by calcitriol (1,25-dihydroxycholecalciferol) excess. Even 1% decrease of calcium reabsorption can provoke hypercalciuria [4]. Hypercalciuria affects from 20% up to 40% of systemic S [5, 6], and up to 50% of patients will develop hypercalciuria at some time during the course of the disease [6]. JA Lancina Martín et coll observed in a retrospective Spanish cohort (96 consequent S patients from 1978 to 1993) hypercalciuria in 26.6% of patients with S and urinary lithiasis or lithogenic risk factors (hypercalcemia and hypercalciuria) [5]. PR Studdy et coll in a UK series, found hypercalciuria in 40% (77 of 192), taking an upper limit of urinary calcium excretion as 300 mg/24 h (7.5 mmol/24 h) [6]. In some past work, hypercalciuria, defined with a lower limit of urinary calcium >200 mg/24 h, was found in 62% of patients [4]. Hypercalciuria often remains asymptomatic, and it

Without renal failure	With renal failure
• Hypercalciuria • Hypercalcemia • Nephrolithiasis • Granulomatous interstitial nephritis • Tubular dysfunction	• Hypercalcemia • Calcium-phosphate deposition and nephrocalcinosis • Tubulous Interstitial nephritis without granulomas (TIN) • Granulomatous interstitial nephritis (rarely) • Glomerular diseases with immune complex deposition • Renovascular disease • Obstructive uropathy

Table 1.
S-associated renal involvements (SARI) and renal failure.

can be remains undiagnosed without hypercalcemia or nephrolithiasis. This could be dangerous because hypercalciuria is a risk factor for nephrolithiasis.

3.2 Frequency of hypercalcemia

In general population, hypercalcemia occurs in 0.2–4%, of which primary hyperparathyroidism and malignancies represent about 80–90% of all cases [7]. Mild to severe hypercalcemia affects from 4% up to 18% of S patients [6, 8]. In the multicenter prospective study ACCESS (a case–control etiologic study of S) [8], R. Baughman and colleagues observed a low frequency of S-associated hypercalcemia 3.7% (27 of 736), perhaps for a 44% of representation of African-Americans where S-associated hypercalcemia is less common. In the ACCESS study, a significant risk factor for S-associated hypercalcemia found (odds ratio 3.6, over 470 patients analyzed) was the combination of HLA DRBI1*1101 allele and exposure to insecticides [9]. Hypercalcemia frequency was 6.3% (6 of 96) in J.A. Lancina Martín's retrospective Spanish cohort [5], whereas P.R. Studdy and colleagues in their UK series found hypercalcemia in 18% (99 of 547, taking an upper limit of normal of 10.5 mg/dl, 2.6 mmol/l) [6]. Referring to the biggest last studies with more than 1000 S patients, hypercalcemia frequency varies from 5 to 11%: In J. Werner's study on Sweden cohort of 1229 S patients (data between 1987 and 2018 collected in local registry at Karolinska University Hospital, Stockholm), 5.4% (66/1229) had hypercalcemia (defined as serum ionized calcium >1.33 mmol/L, reference n.v. 1.15–1.33 mmol/L) [10]. In a single-center retrospective study by R. Baughman and colleagues (n = 1606) reported that hypercalcemia appeared in about 6% of S patients [11]. In this study, a group of about 100 patients with hypercalcemia was compared to 1500 patients with S without calcium metabolism disturbances: there were not any differences in sex, age or ethnicity. In a world survey, James and colleagues noted hypercalcemia in 11% (200/1760) of S patients [12].

3.3 Hypercalcemia in renal sarcoidosis

Hypercalcemia in renal S had a very high prevalence, between 20 and 30%. In A.R. Berliner's meta-analysis [13], the widest sGIN-AKI retrospective study, 19,5% (18/94) of patients were hypercalcemic, 7.7% (4/52) had hypercalciuria, calcitriol was elevated only in one case (1/10), that presented concomitant hypercalcemia. Three patients presented hypercalcemia and inappropriately normal calcitriol. M. Mahévas and colleagues observed a 32% (15/47) hypercalcemia frequency in their retrospective study of the French sarcoidosis Group [14]: hypercalcemia was significantly more common in white patients (44%, 14/32) than in blacks (6.5%, 1/14) (Odd ratio (OR) 8; 95% confidence interval [IC], 1.75–85, $p < 0.001$) and was more common in men than in women (12 vs. 3). There was a seasonal variation of hypercalcemia that is aggravated by sunlight: 50% (11/22) patients diagnosed between June and September had hypercalcemia, compared with only 16% (4/25) patients diagnosed during the other months (OR 7.8; 95% IC, 1.6–44.8, $p < 0.001$). All patients with hypercalcemia presented hypercalciuria, which was complicated by nephrolithiasis in three cases and nephrocalcinosis in one case.

3.4 Frequency of nephrolithiasis

Nephrolithiasis is a complication that happens in 10–14% of S patients over the course of disease, more frequently than in the general population. In A.R. Berliner's meta-analysis 2.7% of S patients have asymptomatic stones at the diagnosis, whereas in 1% of S patients, renal-ureteral colic is the first symptom of disease [13].

Urolithiasis frequency was 14.5% (14/96) in J.A. Lancina Martín's retrospective Spanish cohort with S patients with lithogenic risk factors (hypercalcemia and hypercalciuria) [5].

3.5 Hypercalcemia in sarcoidosis and the role of extrarenal calcitriol

In 1939 for the first time, Harrell and Fisher found an association between dysregulated calcium homeostasis and S granulomas [15]. In the late 1970s, there were observed increased calcitriol concentrations in a few cases of hypercalcemic S patients [16]. In 1981 Barbour and colleagues proved the extrarenal production of activated vitamin D through the observation of hypercalcemia and elevated calcitriol levels in an anephric S patient [17]. In 1982 hypercalcemia and elevated calcitriol levels were observed in a chronic hemodialysis patient with S [18]. Physiologically renal proximal tubular cells transform 25-hydroxycholecalciferol (calcidiol) into 1,25-dihydroxycholecalciferol (calcitriol) through 1-α hydroxylase enzyme. This is under PTH control, which is suppressed by hypercalcemia [19]. Calcitriol is an active vitamin D that increases calcemia, both increasing calcium absorption from bowel and releasing calcium from the bone through the induction of osteoclast cells. It was proved that calcitriol was a metabolite causing S-associated hypercalcemia, and its extrarenal source was found both in activated pulmonary macrophage [20, 21] and in lymph node homogenates [22]. Subsequent works revealed that calcitriol synthesis macrophages are permitted thanks to expression of a single gene, the CYP27B1, and its product 1α-hydroxylase [23]. This extrarenal ectopic production of calcitriol is resistant to negative feedback of hypercalcemia because it is PTH-independent [24]. Many studies confirmed that a high proportion of hypercalcemic S patients have elevated calcitriol [25–27]. The typical pattern of hypercalcemia in S is associated with high plasmatic calcium levels, low intact PTH, and high calcitriol, as observed in the case of AKI due to sGIN presented by Berliner (calcemia 12.9 mg/dl, calciuria 232 mg/24 h, PTH 5.0 pg./ml, calcidiol 38 ng/ml, and calcitriol 120 pg./ml) [13]. In Mahévas's study, 7 of 10 hypercalcemic patients with PTH tested had PTH < 10 ng/l, lower than normal range (n.v. 10–65 ng/l); 7 of 9 hypercalcemic patients with calcidiol tested had calcidiol <10 nmol/L, lower than normal range (n.v. 10–40 nmol/L) [14]. Sometimes calcitriol is in normal range in S patients with hypercalcemia or hypercalciuria, although it is inappropriately normal, and it should be lower in case of hypercalcemia [28]. PTH-related protein, expressed in S granulomas, is another mediator of S-associated hypercalcemia. High series PTH-related protein level was observed in hypercalcemic S patients [29].

4. Diagnosis of renal sarcoidosis

4.1 Frequency of renal sarcoidosis

According to ACCESS Research Group, kidney involvement in S is "unusual but clinically important" [30]. There are various data about frequency of RS, because it depends on what definition is adopted. Considering patients with acute or chronic S, renal involvement is not frequent, as it emerges from geo-epidemiological big data approach to S: in 2019 a review collected large series (>100 patients) of S reported in the PubMed library in the last 20 years, renal involvement frequency was observed in 0.3% patients in Northern Europeans (6/2209 patients with extrathoracic S (ET-S), total patients 71,566), 1.8% patients in Southern European cohorts (26/1477 ET-S patients, total patients 5902), 1.1% patients in US cohorts (28/2436 ET-S patients, total patients 7263), 3.5% patients in Japanese cohorts (36/1027 ET-S patients, total patients 3315) [31].

If RS was interpreted as kidney involvement in S with renal failure, frequency is below 2% of cases: 0.7% (5 of 736) patients of ACCESS study, RS defined as "treatment responsive renal failure" or "steroid-responsive renal failure in a patient with diabetes and/or hypertension" [30]; 1.2% (10 of 818) S patients series of Royal Northern Hospital of London [32].

R. Bergner and colleagues in their German cohort of 327 S patients precisely distinguish between a probable RS and a definite RS [33]:

A patient has a probable RS if two inclusion criteria are satisfied:

- The diagnosis of S according to international guidelines as the American Thoracic Society (ATS) recommendations [34]
- At least one of three renal abnormalities: estimated glomerular filtration rate (eGFR) < 60 ml/min without an alternative explanation, proteinuria >300 mg/g creatinine or > 300 mg/24 h, or abnormal urinary sediment.

A patient has a definite RS if he has a probable RS with a compatible renal histopathology. According to these criteria, frequency of probable and definitive RS is high, respectively, 33.3% (109/327) and 27.5% (90/108) in German cohort. This observation clearly points out how RS is underestimated because asymptomatic in most of cases.

4.2 Pathological urinary sediment and renal sarcoidosis suspect

In A.R. Berliner's meta-analysis at exordium 30% of RS patients had sterile pyuria, 20% hypercalcemia and microhematuria, 10% hypercalciuria and glycosuria [13]. There are not unanimous observation about urinary sediments: In R. Bergner's German cohort 52% renal S patients had pathological sediment (53 of 102 with available sediment, total of 109 patients) in comparison with 29% (51 of 175) S patients without renal involvement (175 patients with available sediment, total 197 patients, $p < 0.001$), difference remained significant observing leukocyturia, more present in renal S patients than in S patients without renal involvement (34%, 37/109 vs. 25%, 43/175, $p < 0.001$) [33]. For R. Bergner and colleagues, pathological urinary sediment was an important tool to identify probable RS.

4.3 Renal biopsy, a fundamental diagnostic tool

Renal biopsy (RBx) can not only identify a further localization of a disease already diagnosed in other organs by biopsy specimens but often manages to give the diagnosis of S, both with systemic involvement since then unknown or with exclusive renal involvement. RS mostly occurs at the presentation of S: in 81% (38/47) in Mahévas's French series [14] and 77% (30/39) in F. Rastelli's Italian series [35]. In Italian series, only four patients (10%, 4/39) had renal S during a systemic disease lasting for more than 1 year, and five patients (13%, 5/39) had exordium symptoms less than 12 months before from RBx. These data were confirmed by Tao Zhao's Beijing cohort, and kidney involvement was the first symptom of S in 83.3% of cases [36]. S diagnosis was possible thanks to renal biopsy in 47% (8/17 patients) in Rajakariar's monocentric study in London [37] and 49% (23/47 patients) in Mahévas's multicentric French study [14]: these patients had an unexplained renal impairment and were subsequently diagnosed with RS involvement and systemic disease. Rastelli and colleagues noticed that RBx permitted the diagnosis of unknown S in 74% (29/39) of Italian patients, whereas in 23% (9/39) of cases presented isolated kidney S. Unexpectedly, 44% (8/18) patients with S lung at diagnosis were without respiratory symptoms, that is 21% (8/39) of patients in Italian series. Not always lung involvement gives rise to dry cough, a frequent symptom in S patients [35]. R. Bergner's and colleagues demonstrated in their German cohort that RBx is a precious diagnostic tool when performed in patients with high suspected renal S: 327 S patients were collected, 109 with probable or definite renal S were identified, of which 72 patients (66%) had eGFR <60mml/min, 57 patients (52%) had proteinuria >300 mg/24 h, 53 patients (49%) had pathological sediment (leukocyturia), in 108 patients RBx was performed, and 90 had confirmed renal S because they had compatible histopathology (sGIN, TIN, nephrolithiasis, and nephrocalcinosis). So RS was confirmed in 83% of cases (90 of 108 RBx performed) [33].

4.4 Phenotypes of renal sarcoidosis patients

In German cohort [33], patients with renal S had more extrapulmonary lymph nodes than other S patients [40% (44/109) vs. 26% (52/197), $p < 0.05$] and more liver involvement [25% (27/109) vs. 16% (31/197), $p = 0.07$].

Clinical phenotype of Mahévas's patients did not differ significantly from patients without renal involvement according to the prevalence of thoracic and extrathoracic localizations [14], similar to the ones in ACCESS study [30].

4.5 Timing for renal biopsy

In the current clinical practice, a patient with systemic S can reach the nephrologist's attention in these two main situations: an impaired renal function with no evidence of decreased kidney perfusion or obstruction and significant proteinuria >1 g/24 h, 2 conditions where there is indication of renal biopsy. Prevalence of renal S is underestimated because only in centers with great expertise in S management RBx is performed in all patients with a suspected renal S: not only in case of decreased renal function or significant proteinuria but even pathological urinary sediment, as R. Bergner and colleagues carried out in their tertiary care centers of German cities of Darmstadt, Géttingen, Ludwigshafen, Offenbach, Trier [33]. To our knowledge, this German multicentric casistic is the widest study of RS for RBx performed.

An impaired renal function can occur with these three clinical conditions: (1) acute kidney injury (AKI): rapidly elevated serum creatinine or an increase, (2) acute kidney injury superimposed on chronic kidney diseases (CKD), and (3) progression of chronic kidney diseases without other leading nephropathogenic causes.

AKI frequency due to RS is low: 0.76% according to Shas's monocenter study considering all 2780 native kidney biopsies performed in The Ohio State University in 7 years, from January 1, 2003 to December 31, 2009: only 21 patients presented a biopsy-proven S with AKI [38]. On the contrary, considering cohort of S patients and not the general population, AKI is not a rare S presentation. In Tao Zhao's cohort in Beijing, kidney involvement was the first symptom of S in 83.3% of cases, with half of them presenting with acute kidney injury [36]. In German cohort two-thirds of patients with renal S histologically confirmed had an eGFR<60 ml/min [33]. R. Bergner and colleagues [33] demonstrated that in patients with systemic S a reduced eGFR below 60 is mainly caused by renal manifestation of disease than other causes: among 109 patients with suspected renal S, renal S was confirmed in 83% of cases

(90 cases of renal S in 108 RBx performed, with interstitial nephritis with or without granulomas in about two-thirds of the patients), wherein only 17% (18/108) there were renal findings not compatible with S: 10.2% (11/108) nephroangiosclerosis, 2.8% (3/108) diabetic nephropathy, 0.9% (1/108) tubular damage, and 2.8% (3/108) unremarkable.

4.6 Severe AKI

In Tao Zhao's cohort in Beijing, 11/18 patients (61.1%) suffered from severe renal function impairment (eGFR <30 mL/min/1.73) at the time of the renal biopsy [36], similar to 68.5% reported in Mahévas's study [14]. The most frequent causes of AKI in RS are hypercalcemia, sGIN, TIN or an association between hypercalcemia with interstitial nephritis in patients suffering from renal sarcoidosis could appear both as sGIN and TIN without granulomas. If hypercalcemia is only a SARI without a disease presence in renal parenchyma, the AKI associated to hypercalcemia is functional and it can be completely recovered. Hypercalcemia provokes a prerenal AKI through a reversible hemodynamic insult due to afferent arteriolar vasoconstriction, hence a decrease in renal blood flow and glomerular filtration rate. If this condition is prolonged, it can cause polyuria and dehydration for inhibition of sodium-potassium ATPase in tubular cell and urinary sodium wasting or tubular necrosis [39].

4.7 Necessity of acute hemodialysis at renal onset

Considering Berliner's meta-analysis, 7,4% of patients (7/94) underwent hemodialysis as acute renal replacement therapy initially or shortly after onset despite steroids.

5. Granulomatous interstitial nephritis in sarcoidosis and other diseases

5.1 sGIN frequency

Sarcoid granulomatous interstitial nephritis (sGIN) is the typical renal lesion in S. Not all sGIN mean have a renal S clinically symptomatic: in fact, it is a silent finding observed at autopsy in 7-23% of S patients [40, 41]. sGIN is mainly observed at RBx performed in the case of AKI, occurring in <1% of S patients [42]. This explains its low frequency, which varies from 0.1 to 0.2% considering the widest American monocentric cohorts of about 10,000 native kidney biopsies performed in 10 year-period up to 1–5% considering RBx in patients referring to tertiary S centers: 0.1% (11/9779) at Harvard Medical School [43], 0.18% (19/10,023) at Johns Hopkins University [44], 1.1% (2/187) in American S cohort at a tertiary S referral center in Minnesota (consecutive patients diagnosed between March 2015 and May 2019), 5% (11/218) Spanish S cohort at tertiary teaching Hospital Clinic of Barcelona (consecutive patients diagnosed between 1990 and 2015) [45]. The epidemiological Japanese study confirmed the low frequency of 0.11% (16/14,191) [46]. sGIN frequency is 0.6% of renal transplant biopsies [47].

5.2 Differential diagnosis of GIN

In relation to N.Joss's study in Glasgow, all causes of GIN represent 1% of all diagnoses on native renal biopsies [48]. According to V.Bijol's study, drug represents

GIN due to all causes	Bijol [43]	Javaud [42]	Joss [48]
Drug	45% (17/38)	17.5% (7/40)	11% (2/18)
S	29% (11/38)	50% (20/40)	28% (5/18)
Wegeners granulomatosis	15.9% (6/38)	2 (5%)	0
idiopathic	10.5% (4/38)	12.5% (5/40)	50% (9/18)
TB	0	7.5% (3/40)	0
Leprosy	0	2.5% (1/40)	0
Mycobacterium avium infection	0	1 (2.5%)	0
Crohn	0	1 (2.5%)	0
foreign-body giant cell reaction	15.9% (6/38)	0	0
bacillus Calmette-Guérin therapy for bladder cancer	15.9% (6/38)	0	0
xanthogranulomatous pyelonephritis	15.9% (6/38)	0	0
TINU syndrome	0	0	11% (2/18)

Table 2.
GIN due to all causes.

the most frequent cause of GIN (45%, 17/38), whereas S is the 2° cause (29%, 11/38) [43], that is to say, that only one out of three cases of GIN is an sGIN (**Table 2**).

In Tao Zhao's cohort in Beijing, sGIN has double frequency (66%, 12/18) respect GIN by other causes (33%, 6/18) [36].

Not caseous non-necrotizing granulomas are typical for RS but not pathognomonic. Many diseases cause GIN, so renal S remain a probability diagnosis. In presence of granuloma physician is more confident of diagnosis of RS, but to have a "definite" diagnosis there are to be excluded all causes of granulomatous inflammation:

- Infectious diseases: brucellosis, fungal infections (histoplasmosis), tuberculosis, and leprosy,
- occupational diseases: chronic beryllium exposure/berylliosis,
- immune-related disease: Crohn's disease, primary Stevens–Johnson syndrome, IgG4-related TIN,
- autoimmune diseases: vasculitis as granulomatosis with polyangiitis, autoimmune-induced TIN,
- reaction due to neoplasm: in particular breast cancer, lung cancer, Hodgkin lymphoma,
- granulomatous foreign-body reaction: heroin, cholesterol atheroembolism, and
- drug-induced interstitial nephritis: nonsteroidal anti-inflammatory drugs, allopurinol, fluoroquinolone antibiotics, diuretics, HIV-antiretroviral, and alfa-interferon.

Other two diseases provoking GIN which are considered as two distinct entities are tubulointerstitial nephritis and uveitis (TINU) syndrome and necrotizing sarcoid granulomatosis (NSG).

5.2.1 Drug-induced interstitial nephritis

Drug-induced interstitial nephritis is the most frequent cause of GIN [49] and it gives rise to interstitial granulomas in 25–50% of cases [50].

The discovery of interstitial granulomas in patients with recent drug intake orients diagnosis toward drug-induced GIN, especially when eosinophils are not present in inflammatory infiltrate [50, 51]. To rule out classical drug-induced interstitial nephritis is important not only an accurate pharmacological anamnesis but also to identify the area interested in granulomatous interstitial reaction: it is the cortical-medullary junction for classical drug-induced interstitial nephritis whereas only renal cortex in sGIN [13, 40].

5.2.2 Tuberculosis

Distinguishing between tuberculosis GIN and sGIN is not always easy in absence of caseous necrosis, typical of tuberculosis and not present in S. Epithelioid not-necrotizing granulomas can be present also in renal tuberculosis. So it is mandatory to recognize Koch bacillum at Ziehl-Neelsen staining and to undertake TB cultures. Polymerase chain reaction (PCR) test of the biopsy for mycobacterial DNA manages to detect Koch bacillum in 67% of cases [52].

Unfortunately, a negative PCR in renal tissue result cannot exclude a TB infection because kidney involvement in TB is not always direct but also indirect, via immune-mediated pathways [53]. E. Danila and E. Zurauskas, demonstrated a significant overlap in types of granulomatous inflammation between tuberculosis and S in the bronchoscopic lung or bronchial biopsies of 105 patients: of patients with tuberculosis, 76% had epithelioid cell granulomas with caseosus necrosis, and 24% had not-necrotizing epithelioid cell granulomas [54].

In **Table 3** there are accuracy characteristics of not-necrotizing granulomas and caseous granulomas, respectively, in diagnosis of S and tuberculosis.

A wrong diagnosis is also a risk in nephrological field: B. Oliveira and colleagues reported four patients who were unnecessarily treated with steroids for an initial

	Sensitivity	Specificity	Positive predictive value	Negative predictive value
Not-necrotizing epithelioid cell granulomas in S diagnosis	94%	60%	68%	92%
epithelioid cell granulomas with caseosus necrosis in tuberculosis diagnosis	76%	85%	69%	88%

Table 3.
Characteristics of not-necrotizing granulomas and caseous granulomas respectively in diagnosis of S and tuberculosis.

diagnosis of renal-limited S (40 mg median dose steroids) and received the right diagnosis of T tuberculosis B infection with a mean delay of 22 months (range: 1–60), one patient before the renal biopsy and three after. All patients at exordium had no evidence of lung tuberculosis, or systemic disease associated with tuberculosis infection, Ziehl Neelson (ZN) stains on the kidney biopsy were negative. Three of these patients extrarenal TB manifestations [55].

Mycobacteria and fungi are the main infective causes of GIN, above all in immunosuppressed patients, such as patients who received renal transplants [47, 56].

5.2.3 Leprosy

Leprosy, provoked by infection with either *Mycobacterium leprae* or *Mycobacterium lepromatosis*, has a worldwide incidence of 200,000 new cases each year [57]. Aiming to consider leprosy in differential diagnosis of GIN, it is fundamental to examine the prevalence of diseases in the area of interest, since 80% of new cases are reported in Brazil, India, and Indonesia [57]. The most frequent kidney involvement in leprosy is amyloidosis [42], whereas GIN is observed only in 1% of leprosy [58].

5.2.4 Fungal infections

Chronic fungal infections have to be ruled out both clinically and through fungal stains on suspected granulomas, such as Grocott-Gomori's methenamine silver stains. In addition, serologic tests should be done in patients living in or coming from endemic areas for *Histoplasma capsulatum* and *Coccidioides immitis*.

In immunodepressed patients with chronic fungal infections, granulomas could present a "dirty" necrosis, characterized by cellular debris and neutrophilic infiltrate, mostly observed in liver during autopsy.

5.2.5 Granulomatosis with polyangiitis

Granulomatosis with polyangiitis (GPA) was also known as Wegener granulomatosis. This vasculitis gives GIN in 5% of cases [59]: the main feature leading to diagnosis is the pauci-immune crescentic glomerulonephritis associated. GPA and S could share some common mechanisms in pathogenesis: some patients presenting with GPA kidney involvement at diagnosis of vasculitis developed biopsy-confirmed lung S months later through cyclophosphamide therapy [60].

Necrotizing sarcoid granulomatosis.

NSG is a condition first described in 1973 by Averill Liebow in the James Burns Amberson lecture to American Thoracic Society. This condition has three main characteristics [61]:

- Histologically: presence of Sarcoid-like granulomas with vasculitis and necrosis.
- Radiologically: multiple lung nodules without hilar adenopathy.
- Clinically: benign course.

To recognize NSG from an S is fundamental to find out necrotizing aspects of granulomatous flogosis, either large foci of necrosis or small central areas of bland necrosis within granulomas. Besides, granulomatous flogosis has focal vasculitis features, with granulomas intruding on the walls of small arteries. It still remains controversial whether NSG is a variant of S or a distinct entity. Liebow suggested that NSG is a variant of angiocentric granulomatosis; according to this hypothesis, granulomas are sarcoid reactions to necrotizing angiitis. The other hypothesis is that NSG is a manifestation of systemic S with necrotic granulomas and may merge with the entity of nodular S [62].

5.2.6 Tubulointerstitial Nephritis and Uveitis syndrome

TINU syndrome is also called Dobrin syndrome because Dobrin described it for the first time in 1975. TINU syndrome is considered a distinct entity from S because of the absence of hypercalcemia, hypercalciuria and bihilar lymphadenopathy [63]. These patients should be evaluated for Sjőrgren's syndrome [64].

5.2.7 Interstitial nephritis in sarcoidosis patients: not always granulomatous

Considering monocentric cohorts of TIN (all causes), in single-center study In T. Zhao's cohort in Beijing, TIN due to renal S was 57% (30/53): sGIN was 23% (12/53) and 34% (18/53) TIN without granulomas considering all causes-GIN, sGIN was 40% (12/30) and 60% (18/30) TIN without granulomas considering RS patients [36].

Considering monocentric RS cohorts, in sGIN frequency was 33% in Rajakariar's series (13 sGIN and 4 TIN without granulomas out of 39 RS cases) [37].

Considering multicentric RS cohorts, in sGIN frequency was 79% (37/47) in Mahévas's series (10 TIN without granulomas and 37 sGIN, of whom 59%, 22/37, with giant cells, out of 47 RS cases) [14], 79% (31/39) in Rastelli's series (31 sGIN and 5 TIN without granulomas, out of 39 RS cases) [35].

6. Demografic and clinic characteristics of sGIN patients

6.1 Sex

If S has a slight predominance in women (female: male ratio 1.2–1.5:1) [1]: female predominance was in ACCESS study [30], 61% (500/818) were female of S patients series of Royal Northern Hospital of London of Royal Northern Hospital of London [32]. RS has a marked predominance in men: in Bergner's German cohort female were 41% (45/109) [33], in Javaud's French study 60% (12/20) [42]. sGIN is more frequent in male gender: 64% in Berliner meta-analysis [13]. The only cohort with different results is Rajakariar's study, where 53% (9/17) of renal S patients were women: probably the high numbers of patients with Afro-Caribbean origin (53%, 9/17) contributed to this different demography [37].

6.2 AGE of onset

RS, as well as sGIN, is more likely to have a later onset than systemic S: in German cohort 58 years (range 18–86) for renal S onset, 51 years (range 19–85) for S onset [33]. In Berliner meta-analysis, mean age at presentation of 94 patients was 46.9 years (range 11–80, for men 46 year, for women 48.5 year) [13]. Mahévas study, the largest retrospective study (47 patients), documented similar data [14]. In Javaud's study, the mean age at presentation of 20 patients with renal S was 51.8 years (range 29–76) [42].

6.3 AKI due to sGIN

In the Italian series, sGIN-AKI resulted more severe than No-sGIN-AKI [35]. In the Berliner meta-analysis regarding sGIN-AKI onset, renal function at presentation was series creatinine 4.8 mg/dl and urinary proteinuria 1 g/24 h [13]. No one of the large studies observed a correlation between proteinuria level and histological findings [65]; nevertheless, a proteinuria >2.0 g/24 h is associated with a glomerular involvement of S, also in the course of sGIN.

7. Pathological characteristics of renal sarcoidosis at diagnosis

7.1 GIN vs TIN without granulomas pathological features independently of causing disease

In order to characterize pathological lesions of TIN T. Zhao and colleagues created a score for active tubulointerstitial injury (including the degeneration or necrosis of tubular epithelial cells, tubulitis, interstitial edema, inflammatory infiltration, and granuloma formation) and a score for chronic tubulointerstitial injury (including tubular atrophy and interstitial fibrosis). Independently of cause of TIN (patients with or without S), 18 patients with granulomatous TIN had higher scores for acute interstitial injury score than 18 patients with TIN without granulomas [6(4.5–7.0) vs. 4(2.0–6.0) p = 0.001)] but Tao Zhao and colleagues did not observe a higher leukocyturia in granulomatous TIN patients (there was leukocyturia in 28% of patients with granulomatous TIN and in 50% patients with TIN without granulomas, p = 0.103) [36].

7.2 Renal sarcoidosis (sGIN and TIN without granulomas) vs tubulointerstitial nephritis in not S patients

In the Chinese cohort of Beijing, chronic tubulointerstitial lesions and glomerulosclerosis were associated with kidney function impairment (eGFR<30 ml/min) in renal S when RBx was performed: renal S (sGIN and sTIN without granulomas) had more chronic tubulointerstitial lesions than non-S patients (GIN and nongranulomatous TIN) at diagnosis: chronic tubular injury score S patients 2(1.030) vs. not S patients 2(0-20), P = 0.060; chronic interstitial injury score: S patients 1.5 (0-3.0) vs. not S patients 1(0–2.0), p = 0.631. At the contrary, not S patients had total tubulointerstitial injury acute score more higher than S patients: 5(4.0–6.0) vs. 10 (6.0–12.0), P = 0.002, in details acute tubular injury score 2(040) vs. 4(20–6.0), p = 0.008, acute interstitial injury score, 5 (3.0–60) vs. 4 (25–60) p = 0.457 [36].

8. Therapy

8.1 Response to steroid therapy

Most patients were treated with prednisone 1 mg/kg as induction therapy. Steroid tapering is started after 12 months since exordium, and average period of maintenance therapy should be 24 months.

All 5 cases described by Joss improved their renal function with an adequate maintenance therapy (Mean follow-up time: 47.2 months (range from 33 to 86)), all patients [48]. In Rajakariar study, all patients showed beneficial responses to prednisolone within the 1° year. In Rajakariar study, there was no difference in response to treatment between black and nonblack patients [37].

8.2 Other studies show no benign prognosis for sGIN-AKI

In the Berliner meta-analysis, most patients improved their renal function but did not regain normal creatinine and were at varying degrees of CKD [13]. In their retrospective study collected 40 cases of GIN due to all causes, Javaud and colleagues observed that sGIN had one of the worse renal function recoveries through steroid therapy other GIN forms because only 65% sGIN patients (13/20) increased renal function after steroid therapy, in comparison with 86% (6/7) drug-induced patients and 100% (5/5) idiopathic GIN. All four patients with Mycobacterium tuberculosis and avium-related GIN and the patient with M. leprae-related GIN recovered their renal function after specific therapy. In the Javaud study, two patients had worse renal function (one patient received a kidney graft after a transient period on hemodialysis), and another with chronic insufficiency died after 3 months of follow-up [42]. In Mahévas study, a complete response to steroids at 1 year was found to be strongly correlated with the complete response at 1 month ([OR] 7; 95% [CI], 1.6-44.8, $p < 0.001$). Furthermore, a complete response to steroids at the end of FU was found to be strongly related to a complete response at 1 month ([OR] 7.6; 95% [CI], 2-41, $p < 0.001$). In Mahévas cases, patients who received high intravenous doses of methylprednisolone (MP) before oral prednisone seem to have a better response to therapy: patients receiving MP had complete response in 80% (8/10), and at the end of follow-up 50%(5/10) had eGFR>60 ml/min, compared to 30%(10/36) patients only receiving oral prednisone [14].

Rajakariar [37] hypercalcemia was strongly correlated with the complete response at 1 year ([OR] 16; 95% [CI], 1.8-137, $p = 0.003$). In a multivariate analysis, hypercalcemia was independently correlated with complete response ($OR = 18.9$, $p = 0.001$).

8.3 Better response for No-sGIN-AKI

In Rajakariar's study, 75% (3/4) of patients with tubulointerstitial nephritis without granulomas, normal calcemia and extrarenal S had steroid-responsive course although advanced scarring at RBx [37]. Rastelli and colleagues confirmed these observations: all 5 No-sGIN-AKI patients had a complete response, independently of histological findings [35].

8.4 Induction with steroid-sparing agent

In Chinese cohort, the five patients who received induction therapy with steroids and steroid-sparing immunosuppressive agents had better long-term kidney recovery than those treated with steroids alone (changes in eGFR%: +221% vs. + 49%, $p = 0.045$) [36]. In German cohort, 35% of patients (38/109) received azathioprine, 4.5% (5/109), mycophenolate mofetil 6.4%, (7/109) methotrexate, unfortunately, outcomes are not available [33].

9. Prognosis (renal outcome and overall survival)

9.1 Pathological prognostic and predictive factors

Rajakariar [37] and Mahévas [14] observed, respectively, 24% (4/17) and 21% (10/47) patients with tubulointerstitial nephritis (TIN) without granulomas. TIN without granulomas patients have a similar response to steroid therapy than in sGIN patients. For authors, this is likely to be due to sampling effect (sparse granulomas are missed in biopsy specimens). Rajakariar [37] recognizes a further factor in advanced disease at presentation. T. Zhao and colleagues found had chronic tubular lesions as a negative predictive response factor independently of the presence of granulomas in interstitial nephritis: renal S patients with satisfactory response at 1 month had chronic tubular injury score significantly lower than S patients who unsatisfactory response: 2(0.5–20) vs. 3(2.0–3.0), p = 0.044 (satisfactory response defined as eGFR increase percent-age > 50% at 1 month after immunosuppression start). Interesting trend showed acute lesions (both tubular and interstitial) as positive predictive response factors.

Renal S patients with satisfactory response at 1 month had both acute tubular injury score and acute interstitial injury score higher than S patients who had unsatisfactory response, even if without statistical significance: respectively 4(2.5–5.5) vs. 1(0–2.0), p = 0.069 and 3(20–40) vs. 3(2.0–4.5), p = 0.930 [36]. Giant cells were present in 59% (22/37) cases of the sGIN Mahévas study [14] and in all five patients of Joss study [48]. There was no relationship between eGFR at 1 month, 1 year and the end of FU and giant cells presence in Mahévas study [14]. Mahévas [14] and colleagues did not find a correlation between the score of granulomas and calcemia [14]. There was no evidence in the literature that granulomas with distinct lymphocyte cuffs around had different prognoses than "naked" granulomas. Five patients in Rajakariar's study [37] had evidence of intracellular calcification. The presence of intracellular calcification was not associated with differences in either presenting renal function or response to corticosteroids. In Mahévas's [14] study, there was interstitial calcification in 8 patients, all with hypercalcemia. There was no relationship between eGFR at 1 month, 1 year and the end of FU and interstitial calcification. In Rajakariar's study [37], there was no correlation between presenting creatinine and the degree of tubular atrophy (Spearman's r = 0.045, P=NS). All patients had tubular fibrosis at biopsy. Final Mean eGFR at 1° year was independent of tubulointerstitial fibrosis degree. Both in Rajakariar [37] and in Mahévas [14] study, interstitial fibrosis was observed in all cases. In Mahévas study, there was an inverse relationship between response to steroids and the initial degree of interstitial fibrosis: patients with low scores of fibrosis were the ones who had the best improvement of renal function, and patients with high scores of fibrosis did not respond to therapy. So interstitial fibrosis is the only pathological finding that correlates with renal outcome. It is a paradox that renal fibrosis is observed in all patients, even in one diagnosis of kidney S is got at disease presentation, for Mahévas renal granulomas should promote fibrosis development very rapidly [14]. In their wider casistic, T. Zhao and colleagues confirmed Mahévas's hypothesis: independently of the cause of GIN (patients with or without S), patients with granulomatous TIN had lower scores for acute tubular injury (p = 0.024) and higher scores for glomerulosclerosis (p = 0.014) and acute interstitial inflammation (p = 0.001) than patients with TIN without granulomas [36].

9.2 Development of CKD

In Berliner meta-analysis, repeated kidney biopsies in patients with bad renal outcomes after steroid therapy showed increased interstitial fibrosis as CKD sign, and some patients progressed toward end-stage kidney disease [13].

Tao Zhao and colleagues noticed that two patients who underwent repeat renal biopsy after 3 months of immunosuppressive treatment showed significant chronic changes coupled with a decreased number of interstitial granulomas, suggesting that immunosuppressive therapies might affect macrophage polarization and thus alter the disease course. In one patient in this study, 3-month immunosuppressive therapy led to the disappearance of renal interstitial M1 macrophages in the kidney biopsy, combined with a good treatment response, thus indicating the potential value of M1 macrophage evaluation in disease monitoring [36].

9.3 ESRD

Since the '80 of last centuries, there have been reports of sGIN patients who had chronic renal failure [66, 67]. Rajakariar's study, one patient was lost to follow-up after 11 years and stopped therapy, subsequently presenting ESRD [37]. One patient in Javaud series reached ESRD and received a kidney graft after a transient period on hemodialysis [42]. In Mahévas's series, 4% of patients who developed end-stage renal disease with S-related disease required initiation of renal replacement therapy (RRT) within 6 months of diagnosis [14]. T. Zhao and colleagues noticed that patients with glomerular involvement showed worse kidney outcomes, with two patients progressing to end-stage renal disease and requiring maintenance hemodialysis [36].

9.4 Relapses

In five patients of Joss's study, relapse occurred in four patients when prednisolone was reduced, and all responded to an increased steroid dose. Three patients of whom were subsequently treated with azathioprine as a steroid-sparing agent. Three of the five patients with S developed extrarenal disease: Granulomas were identified in nasal mucosa in one patient, in lymph node in another patient whereas third patient developed uveitis and restrictive lung defect during follow-up [48]. In Rajakariar's study, 18% (3 of 17) patients relapsed with renal function worsening after stopping steroids because of their side effects or poor compliance, which was reversed upon restarting steroids. Another two patients had multiple relapses as evidenced by AKI and got a complete response with mycophenolate mofetil and azathioprine, respectively, as steroid-sparing agents [37].

In Mahévas's study, 12 patients had relapses (9 extrarenal and 3 renal), all treated with prednisone and additional immunosuppressive (low-dose methotrexate, azathioprine, and mycophenolate mofetil). In 3 cases with renal relapse, both mycophenolate mofetil (2 cases) and azathioprine (1 case) permitted both remission and steroid reduction. Unfavorable response to steroid at 1° month of FU was related to relapse during the disease progression up to the end of FU ($p = 0.049$). The median duration of relapse treatment was 48 months (range 24-76). Mahévas observed the eGFR at the end of FU of patients with renal relapse was not different from that of patients without renal relapses. Rajakariar pointed out that in advanced renal disease, steroid discontinuation appears to lead worsening of renal function, which may reach ESRD [14]. Twenty-eight percent (11/39) of patients in the Italian study had relapses [35]:

nine sGIN-AKI patients, one No-sGIN-AKI patient, and one patient with sGIN and nephrotic syndrome at exordium. Thirteen percent of sGIN-AKI patients (4/31) had another AKI post-RBx. For two patients, AKI occurred after steroid stop (respectively 2 years and 3 months). For the other two patients, AKI occurred on steroid maintenance (respectively during 1° and 3° steroid therapy year). Among nine sGIN-AKI patients with relapse, a patient with isolated renal S had a renal recurrence 2 years later RBx.

9.5 Mortality

Pilar Brito-Zerón and colleagues demonstrated in their Barcelona 218 S cohort that 11 patients with renal involvement had a higher risk of acute complications and increased mortality rates than patients with other extrapulmonary involvement: in fact, between 68 patients with Charlson Comorbidity Index >1 there were patients with a high frequency of RS (8 patients, 11.8%), whereas in 150 patients with Charlson Comorbidity Index (CCI) between 0 and 1 RS was only 2%, three patients ($p = 0.005$). Calcium/vitamin D abnormalities, kidney involvement and death remained significantly associated with a high CCI index after adjusting by age and gender [45]. In an Italian study, three sGIN-AKI patients died during follow-up: one for lung cancer at the age of 85 years, 9 years after RBx; one for pneumonia at the age of 77 years, 6 years after RBx, one for unknown cause at the age of 82 years, 10 years after RBx [35]. In the Javaud study, one patient with renal S and CKD died after 3 months of follow-up [42].

10. Conclusion

The fact that almost 30% of S patients with suspect RS have a real renal involvement makes mandatory a diagnostic renal workout in every patient with a new diagnosis of S. Moreover, RBx should be performed not only in case of renal function impairment but even with urinary abnormalities or proteinuria, since sGIN, in particular, does not have a not benign prognosis. It is fundamental to test whether sGIN-AKI is rapidly responsive to treatment to stop renal fibrosis and avoid AKI transition to CKD. In case of absence of response at 1° line steroid, other immunosuppressors are to be rapidly considered. There are needed RTCs for new drugs. It could be important to know if an early diagnosis, hence a rapid treatment, could affect prognosis.

Acknowledgements

We express great gratitude to ACSI Onlus "Amici contro la Sarcoidosi Italia", the Italian national society of Sarcoidosis patients, in particular to its President Filippo Martoneand the Secretary Amelia Carlucci. ACSI Onlus entirely financed this chapter publication.

Conflict of interest

The authors declare no conflict of interest.

Notes/thanks/other declarations

A particular thanksgiving to Claudia Giuliani.

Author details

Francesco Rastelli*, Luisa Benozzi and Stefano Cusinato
Nephrology and Dialysis, S.S. Trinità Hospital of Borgomanero, Novara, Italy

*Address all correspondence to: fra.rasta83@gmail.com

References

[1] Baughman R, Elyse E, du Bois R. Sarcoidosis. Lancet. 2003;**361**(9363):1111-1118

[2] Garland HG, Thompson JG. Uveo-parotid tuberculosis (Febris uveo-parotidea of heerfordt). QJM: An International Journal of Medicine. 1933;**2**(2):157-178

[3] Adams D. The granulomatous inflammatory response. A review. The American Journal of Pathology. 1976;**84**(1):164

[4] Lebacq E, Verhaegen H, Desmet V. Renal involvement in sarcoidosis. Postgraduate Medical Journal. 1970;**46**(538):526-529

[5] Lancina Martín JA, García Freire C, Busto Castañón L, Picallo Sánchez J, González MM. Sarcoidosis and urolithiasis. Archivos Españoles de Urología. 1995;**48**(3):234-239

[6] Studdy PR, Bird R, Neville E, James DG. Biochemical findings in sarcoidosis. Journal of Clinical Pathology. 1980;**33**(6):528-533

[7] Renaghan AD, Rosner MH. Hypercalcemia: Etiology and management. Nephrology, Dialysis, Transplantation. 2018;**33**(4):549-551

[8] Baughman RP, Teirstein AS, Judson MA, Rossman MD, Yeager H, Bresnitz EA, et al. Clinical characteristics of patients in a case control study of sarcoidosis. American Journal of Respiratory and Critical Care Medicine. 2001;**164**(10 Pt 1):1885-1889

[9] Rossman MD, Thompson B, Frederick M, Iannuzzi MC, Rybicki BA, Pander JP, et al. HLA and environmental interactions in sarcoidosis. Sarcoidosis, Vasculitis, and Diffuse Lung Diseases. 2008;**25**(2):125-132

[10] Werner J, Rivera N, Grunewald J, Eklund A, Iseda T, Darlington P, et al. HLA-DRB1 alleles associate with hypercalcemia in sarcoidosis. Respiratory Medicine. 2021;**187**:106537

[11] Baughman R, Janovcik J, Ray M, Sweiss N, Lower E. Calcium and vitamin D metabolism in sarcoidosis. Sarcoidosis, Vasculitis, and Diffuse Lung Diseases. 2013;**30**(2):113-120

[12] James DG, Neville E, Siltzbach LE, Turiaf J, Battesti JP, Sharma OP, et al. A worldwide review of sarcoidosis. Annals of the New York Academy of Sciences. 1976;**278**(1):321-334

[13] Berliner AR, Haas M, Choi MJ. Sarcoidosis: The nephrologist's perspective. American Journal of Kidney Diseases. 2006;**48**(5):856-870

[14] Mahévas M, Lescure FX, Boffa JJ, Delastour V, Belenfant X, Chapelon C, et al. Renal sarcoidosis: Clinical, laboratory, and histologic presentation and outcome in 47 patients. Medicine. 2009;**88**(2):98-106

[15] Harrell GT, Fisher S. Blood chemical changes IN BOECK'S sarcoid with particular reference to protein, calcium and phosphatase values. The Journal of Clinical Investigation. 1939;**18**(6):687-693

[16] Bell NH, Stern PH, Pantzer E, Sinha TK, DeLuca HF. Evidence that increased circulating 1 alpha, 25-dihydroxyvitamin D is the probable cause for abnormal calcium metabolism

in sarcoidosis. The Journal of Clinical Investigation. 1979;**64**(1):218-225

[17] Barbour GL, Coburn JW, Slatopolsky E, Norman AW, Horst RL. Hypercalcemia in an anephric patient with sarcoidosis: Evidence for extrarenal generation of 1,25-dihydroxyvitamin D. The New England Journal of Medicine. 1981;**305**(8):440-443

[18] Maesaka JK, Batuman V, Pablo NC, Shakamuri S. Elevated 1,25-dihydroxyvitamin D levels: Occurrence with sarcoidosis with end-stage renal disease. Archives of Internal Medicine. 1982;**142**(6):1206-1207

[19] Gardner DG. Hypercalcemia and sarcoidosis--another piece of the puzzle falls into place. The American Journal of Medicine. 2001;**110**(9):736-737

[20] Adams JS, Sharma OP, Gacad MA, Singer FR. Metabolism of 25-hydroxyvitamin D3 by cultured pulmonary alveolar macrophages in sarcoidosis. The Journal of Clinical Investigation. 1983;**72**(5):1856-1860

[21] Adams JS, Gacad MA. Characterization of 1 alpha-hydroxylation of vitamin D3 sterols by cultured alveolar macrophages from patients with sarcoidosis. The Journal of Experimental Medicine. 1985;**161**(4):755-765

[22] Mason RS, Frankel T, Chan YL, Lissner D, Posen S. Vitamin D conversion by sarcoid lymph node homogenate. Annals of Internal Medicine. 1984;**100**(1):59-61

[23] Ichi TK, Kitanaka S, Sato T, Kobori M, Yanagisawa J, Kato S. 25-hydroxyvitamin D3 1α-hydroxylase and vitamin D synthesis. Science. 1997;**277**(5333):1827-1830

[24] Reichel H, Koeffler P, Barbers R, Norman AW. Regulation of 1,25-Dihydroxyvitamin D3 production by cultured alveolar macrophages from Normal human donors and from patients with pulmonary sarcoidosis. The Journal of Clinical Endocrinology & Metabolism. 1987;**65**(6):1201-1209

[25] Papapoulos SE, Clemens TL, Fraher LJ, Lewin IG, Sandler LM, O'Riordan JL. 1, 25-dihydroxycholecalciferol in the pathogenesis of the hypercalcaemia of sarcoidosis. Lancet. 1979;**1**(8117):627-630

[26] Sharma OP. Vitamin D, calcium, and sarcoidosis. Chest. 1996;**109**(2):535-539

[27] Sharma OP. Hypercalcemia in granulomatous disorders: A clinical review. Current Opinion in Pulmonary Medicine. 2000;**6**(5):442-447

[28] Ponce C, Gujral JS. Renal failure and hypercalcemia as initial manifestations of extrapulmonary sarcoidosis. Southern Medical Journal. 2004;**97**(6):590-592

[29] Zeimer HJ, Greenaway TM, Slavin J, Hards DK, Zhou H, Doery JC, et al. Parathyroid-hormone-related protein in sarcoidosis. The American Journal of Pathology. 1998;**152**(1):17-21

[30] Judson MA, Baughman RP, Teirstein AS, Terrin ML, Yeager H. Defining organ involvement in sarcoidosis: The ACCESS proposed instrument. ACCESS research group. A case control etiologic study of sarcoidosis. Sarcoidosis, Vasculitis and Diffuse Lung Diseases. 1999;**16**(1):75-86

[31] Brito-Zeron P, Kostov B, Superville D, Baughman RP, Ramos-Casals M. Geoepidemiological big data approach to sarcoidosis: Geographical and ethnic determinants. Clinical and Experimental Rheumatology. 2019;**37**(6):1052-1064

[32] James DG. Sarcoidosis. Postgraduate Medical Journal. 1984;**60**(701):234-241

[33] Bergner R, Weiner SM, Kehl G, de Groot K, Tielke S, Asendorf T, et al. Renal disease in sarcoidosis patients in a German multicentric retrospective cohort study. Respiratory Medicine. 2023;**209**:107121

[34] Crouser ED, Maier LA, Wilson KC, Bonham CA, Morgenthau AS, Patterson KC, et al. Diagnosis and detection of sarcoidosis. An official American Thoracic Society clinical practice guideline. American Journal of Respiratory and Critical Care Medicine. 2020;**201**(8):e26-e51

[35] Rastelli F, Baragetti I, Buzzi L, Ferrario F, Benozzi L, Di Nardo F, et al. Renal involvement in sarcoidosis: Histological patterns and prognosis, an Italian survey. Sarcoidosis, Vasculitis, and Diffuse Lung Diseases. 2021;**38**(3):e2021017

[36] Zhao T, Yu X, Wang S, Yang L, Su T. Hypercalciuria may predict better response to immunosuppressive therapy in renal sarcoidosis: A case series. Journal of Nephrology. 2023;**36**(1):69-82

[37] Rajakariar R, Sharples E, Raftery M, Sheaff M, Yaqoob M. Sarcoid tubulo-interstitial nephritis: Long-term outcome and response to corticosteroid therapy. Kidney International. 2006;**70**(1):165-169

[38] Shah R, Shidham G, Agarwal A, Albawardi A, Nadasdy T. Diagnostic utility of kidney biopsy in patients with sarcoidosis and acute kidney injury. International Journal of Nephrology and Renovascular Disease. 2011;**4**:131-136

[39] Benabe JE, Martinez-Maldonado M. Hypercalcemic nephropathy. Archives of Internal Medicine. 1978;**138**(5):777-779

[40] Longcope W, Freiman D. A study of sarcoidosis; based on a combined investigation of 160 cases including 30 autopsies from the Johns Hopkins Hospital and Massachusetts General Hospital. Medicine (Baltimore). 1952;**31**(1):1-132

[41] Ricker W, Clark M. Sarcoidosis; a clinicopathologic review of 300 cases, including 22 autopsies. American Journal of Clinical Pathology. 1949;**19**(8):725-749

[42] Javaud N, Belenfant X, Stirnemann J, Laederich J, Ziol M, Callard P, et al. Renal granulomatoses: A retrospective study of 40 cases and review of the literature. Medicine. 2007;**86**(3):170-180

[43] Bijol V, Mendez GP, Nose V, Rennke HG. Granulomatous interstitial nephritis: A clinicopathologic study of 46 cases from a single institution. International Journal of Surgical Pathology. 2006;**14**(1):57-63

[44] Bagnasco SM, Gottipati S, Kraus E, Alachkar N, Montgomery RA, Racusen LC, et al. Sarcoidosis in native and transplanted kidneys: Incidence, pathologic findings, and clinical course. PLoS One. 2014;**9**(10):e110778

[45] Brito-Zerón P, Acar-Denizli N, Sisó-Almirall A, Bosch X, Hernández F, Vilanova S, et al. The burden of comorbidity and complexity in sarcoidosis: Impact of associated chronic diseases. Lung. 2018;**196**(2):239-248

[46] Kamata Y, Sato H, Joh K, Tsuchiya Y, Kunugi S, Shimizu A, et al. Clinical characteristics of biopsy-proven renal sarcoidosis in Japan. Sarcoidosis, Vasculitis, and Diffuse Lung Diseases. 2018;**35**(3):252

[47] Meehan SM, Josephson MA, Haas M. Granulomatous tubulointerstitial nephritis in the renal

allograft. American Journal of Kidney Diseases. 2000;**36**(4):E27

[48] Joss N, Morris S, Young B, Geddes C. Granulomatous interstitial nephritis. Clinical Journal of the American Society of Nephrology. 2007;**2**(2):222-230

[49] Schwarz A, Krause PH, Keller F, Offermann G, Mihatsch MJ. Granulomatous interstitial nephritis after nonsteroidal anti-inflammatory drugs. American Journal of Nephrology. 1988;**8**(5):410-416

[50] Kleinknecht D, Vanhille P, Druet P. Acute granulomatous interstitial nephritis of drug origin. Presse Médicale. 1988;**17**(5):201-205

[51] Mignon F, Méry JP, Mougenot B, Ronco P, Roland J, Morel-Maroger L. Granulomatous interstitial nephritis. Advances in Nephrology from the Necker Hospital. 1984;**13**:219-245

[52] Agrawal V, Kaul A, Prasad N, Sharma K, Agarwal V. Etiological diagnosis of granulomatous tubulointerstitial nephritis in the tropics. Clinical Kidney Journal. 2015;**8**(5):524-530

[53] Eastwood JB, Corbishley CM, Grange JM. Tuberculosis and tubulointerstitial nephritis: An intriguing puzzle. Kidney International. 2011;**79**(6):579-581

[54] Danila E, Zurauskas E. Diagnostic value of epithelioid cell granulomas in bronchoscopic biopsies. Internal Medicine. 2008;**47**(24):2121-2126

[55] Oliveira B, Jayawardene S, Shah S. Single-Centre experience of granulomatous interstitial nephritis-time for a new approach? Clinical Kidney Journal. 2017;**10**(2):249-254

[56] Gonçalves AR, Caetano MA, Paula FJ, Ianhez LE, Saldanha LB, Sabbaga E. Tuberculous interstitial granulomatous nephritis in renal transplants: Report of three cases. Transplantation Proceedings. 1992;**24**(5):1911

[57] Sugawara-Mikami M, Tanigawa K, Kawashima A, Kiriya M, Nakamura Y, Fujiwara Y, et al. Pathogenicity and virulence of Mycobacterium leprae. Virulence;**13**(1):1985-2011

[58] Nakayama EE, Ura S, Fleury RN, Soares V. Renal lesions in leprosy: A retrospective study of 199 autopsies. American Journal of Kidney Diseases. 2001;**38**(1):26-30

[59] Bajema IM, Hagen EC, van der Woude FJ, Bruijn JA. Wegener's granulomatosis: A meta-analysis of 349 literary case reports. The Journal of Laboratory and Clinical Medicine. 1997;**129**(1):17-22

[60] Ahuja TS, Mattana J, Valderrama E, Sankaran R, Singhal PC, Wagner JD. Wegener's granulomatosis followed by development of sarcoidosis. American Journal of Kidney Diseases. 1996;**28**(6):893-898

[61] Yeboah J, Afkhami M, Lee C, Sharma OP. Necrotizing sarcoid granulomatosis. Current Opinion in Pulmonary Medicine. 2012;**18**(5):493-498

[62] Churg A, Carrington CB, Gupta R. Necrotizing sarcoid granulomatosis. Chest. 1979;**76**(4):406-413

[63] Nzerue C, Schlanger L, Jena M, Hewan-Lowe K, Mitch WE. Granulomatous interstitial nephritis and uveitis presenting as salt-losing nephropathy. American Journal of Nephrology. 1997;**17**(5):462-465

[64] Vidal E, Rogues AM, Aldigier JC. The Tinu syndrome or the Sjögren syndrome? Annals of Internal Medicine. 1992;**116**(1):93

[65] Bergner R, Hoffmann M, Waldherr R, Uppenkamp M. Frequency of kidney disease in chronic sarcoidosis. Sarcoidosis, Vasculitis, and Diffuse Lung Diseases. 2003;**20**(2):126-132

[66] Farge D, Lioté F, Turner M, Barré P, Jothy S. Granulomatous nephritis and chronic renal failure in sarcoidosis. Long-term follow-up studies in two patients. American Journal of Nephrology. 1986;**6**(1):21-27

[67] Tsiouris N, Kovacs B, Daskal I, Brent LH, Samuels A. End-stage renal disease in sarcoidosis of the kidney. American Journal of Kidney Diseases. 1999;**34**(5):E21

Chapter 6

Sarcoidosis and Acute Kidney Injury

Marilena Stoian

Abstract

Sarcoidosis is a multi-organ disease characterized by the formation of non-caseating epithelioid granulomas in many organs. The kidneys are not commonly affected but when the disease involves these organs. It is comprised of non-caseating granulomatous interstitial nephritis (GIN) and hypercalcemia-related disorders. In the latter case, acute kidney injury as initial presentation of the disease is a rare entity, and it is postulated to appear due to several pathogenic processes: (1) interstitial nephritis with or without granulomas, (2) nephrocalcinosis with or without nephrolithiasis, and (3) urethral obstruction. A 71-year-old man presented to the clinic with a history of lethargy, nausea, short memory loss and a 10 kg weight loss all of which appeared within the past 6 months. He was also known with prostate adenoma and was under the care of a urologist. Upon physical examination the following aspects were noted: blood pressure of 160/100 mmHg, heart rate 60 bpm and an irregular enlarged prostate. The chest X-ray was normal and blood samples revealed anemia, hypercalcemia, and increased values of urea and creatinine. An ultrasound of the kidneys was performed and no abnormalities were noted. The urinalysis showed the presence of protein +, glucose+, blood 2+, a few white cells and some granular casts. The next step was to perform a renal biopsy that revealed areas of lymphocytic tubulitis, mild mononuclear interstitial infiltrate, some non-necrotizing epithelioid granulomas comprised of Langerhans-type giant cells and epithelioid macrophages. Peri-tubular interstitial calcifications were also noted. As a result a histological diagnosis was summarized as acute or chronic granulomatous interstitial nephritis with nephrocalcinosis. A CT scan pf the chest was subsequently performed and it revealed calcified lymph nodes in the mediastinum involving the space between the aorta and the trachea and numerous nodules scattered bilateralally over the entire lung parenchyma with no apparent periseptal or perivascular association. These findings were diagnosed as sarcoidosis. The serum ACE level was found abnormal and therefore, a clinical diagnosis of sarcoidosis was made and the patient was started on 40 mg of oral prednisone daily with rapid improvement in the overall general condition. Sarcoidosis is an uncommon disease that should be suspected in front of a patient that presents with hypercalcemia and acute kidney injury. After excluding other causes of hypercalcemia such as multiple myeloma, primary hyperparathyroidism, and paraneoplastic phenomena, a renal biopsy is then indicated to confirm the diagnosis of sarcoidosis.

Keywords: sarcoidosis, hypercalcemia, acute kidney injury, non-caseating granulomatous interstitial nephritis (GIN), nephrocalcinosis

1. Introduction

Sarcoidosis is a rare condition of unknown etiology characterized by systemic inflammation. In more than 90% of patient sarcoidosis mainly involves the respiratory and lymphatic systems [1]. The pathogenesys is not completely understood and it relies on an aberrant T cell response to unidentified antigens together with a genetic predisposition and the effect of environmental factors in predisposed individuals. The hallmark feature of sarcoidosis is the formation of non caseating granulomas in the affected organs. These structures are characterized by increased expression of polarized macrophages together with a defective link between regulator and effector T cells. There is a very complex interplay of immune cells which include macrophages, dendritic cells, T helper lymphocytes, T regulatory cells (Tregs) and their medators [2]. The exact etiologic agent (s) is still unknown although studies of T cell antigen receptor (TCR) Vbeta interactions suggest conventional antigenic stimulation. The most investigated agents are infectious agents (components of cutibacteria and mycobacteria), occupational and environmental exposures, Kveim-Siltzbach reagent and vimentin [3, 4].

Kidney involvement in sarcoidosis is rare and not well understood and it is defined either by histologic changes or just by a decline in kidney function. Several small studies showed that the disease can affect the kidneys in 10 to 50% of the patients [5, 6] and most of the times the disease remains silent or undetected for many years. In a large cohort that included some 1200 patients with pulmonary sarcoidosis kidney disease was detected in 12% of cases [7]. The ACCESS study revealed that renal involvement detected at 6 months after the initial diagnosis was present in only 5 patients (0.7%) out of a total of 736 cases investigated [8].

The main kidney abnormalities in sarcoidosis are noncaseating granulomatous interstitial nephritis (GIN) and hypercalcemia-related disorders, with a difficult clinical diagnosis. With regards to outcome, there is a large variability with some patient that progress to end-stage kidney disease (ESKD) and some that experience spontaneous remision. We now know that early disgnosis and the rapid onset of corticotherapy can improve the prognosis. The acute kidney injury (AKI) is thought to appear by means of hypercalcemia that induces vasoconstriction of the afferent arterioles. The most common causes of hypercalcemia include: hyperparathyroidism, multiple myeloma, bone metastases and humoral hypercalcemia associated with malignancy. Less common causes are sarcoidosis, hyperthyroidism, Addison's disease, drug related hypercalcemia and vitamin D excess. The most prevalent complications are nephrocalcinosis and renal stones. The interstitial nephritis associated with sarcoidosis is suspected in patients who present with an elevated creatinine and a bland urine sediment and have a known diagnostic or a characteristic presentation of extrarenal sarcoidosis. In patients that develop ESKD dialysis and transplantation can offer results similar to those with other causes of kidney failure. Even if renal involvement is a rare occurence in sarcoidosis it can nevertheless influence the prognosis of the disease. It is therefore important to detect early changes in kidney function in order top revent the progression to ESKD.

2. Kidney disease in sarcoidosis

Sarcoidosis by means of the associated inflammation can affect virtually every organ but with a great predisposition for pulmonary involvement. In up to 30% of cases the presentation involves sarcoid lesions in the skin, the eyes, reticuloendothelial and musculoskeletal systems, in the exocrine glands, the heart, the kidneys and the central nervous system.

In a retrospective multicenter study (EpiSarc) that included 562 men and 675 women there were 5 distinct phenotypes of sarcoidosis detected with a non-random distribution of organ involvement [7]. These phenotypes are distinctive by means of sex, geographical origin and socio-professional category:

1. pulmonary involvement with fibrosis and heart involvement (associated with being non-European/non-White)

2. hepatosplenic, peripheral lymph node and bone involvement (associated with being non-European/non-White)

3. erythema nodosum, joint involvement and hilar lymph nodes (associated with being European/White and female)

4. eye, neurological, digestive and *kidney* involvement nodes (associated with being European/White)

5. lupus pernio and a high percentage of severe involvement

In contrast to the EpiSarc an earlier European study of White/ CAUCASIAN patients with sarcoidosis (The Genotype-Phenotype Relationship in Sarcoidosis study) identified five different subgroups:

1. abdominal organ involvement

2. ocular-cardiac-cutaneous-central nervous system (CNS) disease involvement,

3. musculoskeletal-cutaneous involvement,

4. pulmonary and intrathoracic lymph node involvement,

5. extrapulmonary involvement [9].

Kidney involvement in sarcoidosis has not been studied thoroughly. The are several small and larger studies that determined that renal disease occurs in 10–50% of patients with sarcoidosis. The characteristic lesions have different causes and prevalance:

1. **nephrocalcinosis** is estimated to occur in 5% of patients with sarcoidosis [10];

2. **nephrolithiasis** occurs in approximately 1–14% of patients with sarcoidosis [11, 12];

3. **interstitial nephritis** with granuloma formation occurs in approximately 20% of patients [13];

4. **glomerular involvement** include membranous nephropathy, IgA nephropathy, minimal change disease, proliferative or crescentic glomerulonephritis, and focal segmental glomerulosclerosis [14];

5. **urinary tract obstruction** resulting from retroperitoneal lymph node involvement, retroperitoneal fibrosis, kidney stones, and direct ureteral involvement by sarcoid [15];

6. **retroperitoneal fibrosis** involve the renal artery, which may be affected by sarcoid angiitis associated with hypertension [16].

Acute kidney injury (AKI) was detected in 0.7% to 4.3% of patients with sarcoidosis it has several causes: (1) nephrocalcinosis with or without nephrolithiasis, (2) interstitial nephritis with or without granulomas [17] and (3) ureteral obstruction. Acute kidney injury rarely appears as the initial presentation of the disease. To make a correct diagnosis the clinical presentation needs to be combined with paraclinical tests and with renal pathology. The treatment with steroids usually produces a good effect on AKI.

End stage renal disease (ESRD) appears most likely due to hypercalcemic nepropathy rather than granulomatous nephritis or a glomerulonephropathy. This happens in spite of the fact that nephrocalcinosis is less common overall than interstitial nephritis. Risk factors for ESKD included advanced age at the time of kidney disease diagnosis, granulomatous tubulointerstitial nephritis, and interstitial fibrosis [17]. Even though many patients with sarcoidosis and ESKD have a reduced eGFR they rarely require some form of kidney replacement therapy. Sarcoid reccurence in the kidney after renal transplantation has been observed at a median of 13 months after the surgical intervention in 27% of patients and this suggests that specific clinical and histologic monitoring may be warranted during the early post-transplant period [18, 19].

Hypercalcemia represents a well known complication of sarcoidosis and is found in 10 to 20% of patients. It can directly cause acute kidney injury due to renal vasoconstriction and volume depletion as a result of nephrogenic diabetes insipidus [20]. It appears because of hyperproduction of 1,25-dihydroxy vitamin D.. The normal conversion of 25-hydroxyvitamin D (calcidiol) to 1,25-dihydroxyvitamin D (calcitriol) occurs in the kidney through 1-α hydroxylase, a cytochrome p 450 enzyme [21, 22]. In sarcoidosis and other granulomatous diseases pulmonary macrophages express 1-α hydroxylase, which is often resistant to negative feedback mechanisms causing overproduction of calcitriol [21, 23] which in turn leads to increased calcium uptake by the gut. Adams et al. demonstrated that calcitriol is the hypercalcemia-causing factor in sarcoidosis and that macrophages from patients with sarcoidosis are the synthetic source of hormone in the disease [24]. In sarcoid granulomas incubated with 25-hydroxy vitamin D, Mason et al. identified a similar metabolite [25]. It has also been shown that in sarcoidosis but also in other granulomatous conditions, some activated mononuclear cells (particularly macrophages) located in the lungs and lymph nodes can produce calcitriol from calcidiol in a mechanism independent of PTH [24–26]. The evidence for extrarenal calcitriol production is comes from several observations [24–27]:

- hypercalcemia and serum calcitriol concentrations have been described in an anephric patient with sarcoidosis;

- calcidiol conversion to calcitriol can be demonstrated in vitro in alveolar macrophages or lymph node tissue obtained from hypercalcemic patients with sarcoidosis;

- production of the messenger RNA for CYP27B1, the 1-hydroxylase, is markedly increased in alveolar macrophages isolated from hypercalcemic patients with sarcoidosis.

In some patients with sarcoidosis parathyroid hormone-related protein (PTHrP), the usual etiologic agent of humoral hypercalcemia of malignancy, may also contribute to the hypercalcemia. In one series, PTHrP was found in 85% (17 of 20) of biopsies of granulomatous tissue from patients with sarcoidosis, and a few patients with both sarcoidosis and hypercalcemia had high serum PTHrP concentrations [28].

Hypercalciuria is three times more common than hypercalcemia [20] in patients with sarcoid and some studies show a frequency of up to 60% of cases [29]. Even though hypercalciuria appears in 30–60% of patients with sarcoidosis an abnormal calcitriol metabolism is seen in subjects who are normocalciuric and also normocalcemic [30]. In normal people if we increase the calcium intake then we obtain a lowering of serum calcitriol concentration but this does not happen in patients with sarcoidosis.

Both hypercalcemia and hypercalciuria can lead to acute and chronic kidney injury in sarcoidosis by causing nephrolithiasis and nephrocalcinosis. Hypercalcemia by means of preglomerular arterial vasoconstriction may cause a decreased glomerular filtration rate (GFR) [31]. The formation of calcium oxalate crystals is the likely cause of nephrolithiasis and it comes from the interplay between hypercalcemia and hypercalciuria. Interstitial calcium oxalate deposition is also seen in association with granulomas in sarcoidosis [32]. Measurement of serum calcium, 24-hour urinary calcium concentration, and a serum angiotensin-converting enzyme (ACE) concentration may provide support for the diagnosis of sarcoidosis. The causes of hypercalcemia are listed below in **Table 1**. The most frequent are: multiple myeloma, hyperparathyroidism, bone metastases and humoral hypercalcaemia of malignancy. Less common causes include sarcoidosis, Addison s disease and drugs.

The aim of compensatig the hypercalcemia and hypercalciuria associated to sarcoidosis is reducing intestinal calcium absorption and calcitriol synthesis. The main requirements are reducing calcium intake to a maximum of 400 mg per day, reducing oxalate intake, avoidance of sun exposure and eliminating all types of vitamin D supplements. Treatment with glucocorticoids decreases inflammation and therefore calcitriol synthesis while bisphosphonates are used to successfully treat the hypercalcemia. Apart from these,; chloroquine, hydroxychloroquine, and ketoconazole can improve calcium metabolism in patients with sarcoidosis.

Urinary tract obstruction appears in sarcoidosis due to the following factors: Retroperitoneal lymph node involvement, retroperitoneal fibrosis, kidney stones, and direct ureteral involvement by sarcoid. Type AA amyloidosis in association with the characteristic inflammation has been described in the renal biopsy of one patient with systemic sarcoidosis [33]. The renal artery can suffer from sarcoid angiitis also associating hypertension which can also appear due to retroperitoneal fibrosis. All of the above conditions are hallmarks and causes of AKI and may respond to corticosteroids, urologic decompression and hemodialysis [34].

Granulomatous interstitial nephritis (GIN) is one of the lesions that are identified in renal biopsieis in patients with sarcoidosis. It is usually silent but occasionally it may present as acute kidney injury [35]. GIN is encountered in 0.5–0.9% of native renal biopsieis and in 0.6% of renal transplant biopsies [36–39]. However,

I. Parathyroid hormone-related
1. Primary hyperparathyroidism
2. Sporadic, familial, associated with multiple endocrine neoplasia I or II
3. Tertiary hyperparathyroidism
4. Associated with chronic renal failure or vitamin D deficiency
II. Vitamin D-related
1. Vitamin D intoxication
2. Usually 25-hydroxyvitamin D_2 in over-the-counter supplements
3. Granulomatous disease: sarcoidosis, berylliosis, tuberculosis
4. Hodgkin's lymphoma
III. Malignancy
1. Humoral hypercalcemia of malignancy (mediated by PTHrP)
2. Solid tumors, especially lung, head, and neck squamous cancers, renal cell tumors
3. Local osteolysis (mediated by cytokines) multiple myeloma, breast cancer
IV. Medications
1. Thiazide diuretics (usually mild)
2. Lithium
3. Milk-alkali syndrome (from calcium antacids)
4. Vitamin A intoxication (including analogs used to treat acne)
V. Other endocrine disorders
1. Hyperthyroidism
2. Adrenal insufficiency
3. Acromegaly
4. Pheochromocytoma
VI. Genetic disorders
1. Familial hypocalciuric hypercalcemia: mutated calcium-sensing receptor
VII. Other
1. Immobilization, with high bone turnover (e.g., Paget's disease, bedridden child)
2. Recovery phase of rhabdomyolysis

Table 1.
Causes of hypercalcemia.

some 7–27% of patients with sarcoidosis have evidence of granulomatous tubulointerstitial nephritis on post-mortem series, although this may not result in clinically significant renal disease. In a small number of patients with sarcoidosis GIN can precede the diagnostic but as a general rule it is now known that GIN can develop at any time during the course of the disease [40]. There are several causes of granulomatous interstitial nephritis among which are: drugs (cephalosporins, vancomycin, nitrofurantoin, ciprofloxacin and NSAIDs) (9–45%), sarcoidosis (9–29%), mycobacterial or fungal infections, crystal deposits, paraproteinemia, granulomatosis with polyangiitis (GPA), and very rarely inflammatory bowel diseases. GIN also appears as a idiopathic entity (>40%) [13, 41]. The relative contribution of different etiologies to GIN is unknown since our knowledge is based on case series and case reports for the description of this condition. In a report by Mignon *et al.* [42] of 32 cases, ~28% were due to drugs, 16% were caused by granulomatosis with polyangiitis (GPA) and 9% were attributed to sarcoidosis and tuberculosis. Furthermore, in a retrospective of 40 consecutive renal biopsiei where GIN was defined as the presence of at least one epithelioid granuloma in the interstitium, Javaud et al. [40] found that the majority of cases were caused by sarcoidosis (50%), followed by medication induced (17.5%) and tuberculosis associated in 7.5% of cases. Membranous nephropathy can be detected in conjunction with GIN in patients with sarcoidosis with a good response to glucocorticoid therapy [43].

In the granulomas of sarcoidosis,secretion of tumor necrosis factor (TNF) by macrophages is followed by a complex interplay of T helper (Th) 1 and Th17 cells with subsequent synthesis of interleukin-6 (IL-6), IL-12, IL-18, IL-23 and transforming growth factor (TGF)-β [38, 44]. All these cytokines further stimulate the macrophages and lead to functional changes and maturation into epithelioid cells and eventually giant cells [45, 46]. Natural killer (NK) cells are also involved and they produce interferon (IFN)-γ which also promotes inflammation. Glucocorticosteroids exert their beneficial effect on granulomas by repression of NF-κB-related gene transcription with lymphocyte apoptosis [46]. Until recently, the granuloma was seen as a static structure but research in tuberculosis has revealed that these structures are highly dynamic [44]. An improved understanding of granuloma formation and interactions may reveal useful therapeutic targets for the future [44].

Mild proteinuria and/or sterile pyuria can appear in association with the interstitial nephritis but usually the urinalysis looks normal. Significant proteinuria is uncommon. In a review of 52 cases of sarcoidosis interstitial nephritis, sterile pyuria, hematuria, glycosuria, and hypercalciuria were identified in 33, 21, 12, and 8% of cases, respectively [10]. In a prospective review of 191 sarcoid patients, proteinuria, defined as urine protein/creatinine ratio equal to or exceeding 0.3 mg/mg, was found in 7% of cases [47]. More than half of these patients had another known risk factor for proteinuria (diabetes, hepatitis B or C infection, human immunodeficiency virus [HIV], systemic lupus erythematosus, or congestive heart failure).

3. Acute kidney injury -an atipical modality of the onset of sarcoidosis: clinical case

A 71-year-old man presented to the clinic with a 6-months old history of lethargy, nausea, weight loss (10 kg) and short-term memory loss. He was also under urologist observation for a PSA of 34 μg/l (normal range < 4 μg/l) associated with benign prostatic hypertrophy. Upon physical examination it was noted that the patient had a blood pressure of 160/100 mmHg, heart rate pf 60 bpm and an enlarged prostate gland. The chest X ray was normal. Biological examination showed anemia (hemoglobin 10.4 g/dl) with normal range of white and platelet cells, raised serum urea (40 mmol/l) and serum creatinine (680 μmol/l) and also hypercalcaemia (3 mmol/l). There were no antibodies detected suggesting of autoimmune disease. Furthermore the renal ultrasound was normal, urinalysisi showed erythrocytes 2+, protein +, glucose +, a few leucocytes and granular casts. The decision was then to perform a renal biopsy which showed foci of lymphocytic tubulitis and a mild mononuclear interstitial infiltrate; focal peri-tubular interstitial calcification; several discrete non-necrotizing epithelioid granulomata comprised of epitheliod macrophages and Langerhans-type giant cells. The histological diagnosis was then made as acute or chronic granulomatosis interstitial nephritis with nephrocalcinosis (**Figure 1**). The patient was then subjected to a CT scan of the chest which revealed calcified mediastinal lymph nodes between the aorta and the trachea, intra-pulmonary nodules scattered throughout the upper and lower lobes without any apparent perivascular or peri- septal association (**Figure 2**). The native pelvic and abdominat CT scans showed the presence of a non obstructing 3 mm calculus in the left kidney with normal size organs and no nephorcalcinosis (**Figure 3**). The scan findings were consistent with sarcoidosis. The serum ACE level was abnormal (200 U/l – normal range: 27-82 U/l), PTH was low <3 (11–67 pg./mL), also with low serum level of 25-hydroxyvitamin D 23.8 (30–95 ng/mL), but a high level of 1,25-dihydroxyvitamin D 79 (18–72 pg./mL). A clinical diagnosis of sarcoidosis was made and the patient was started on 40 mg prednisone /day orally. A rapid improvement of the patient's condition was then noted.

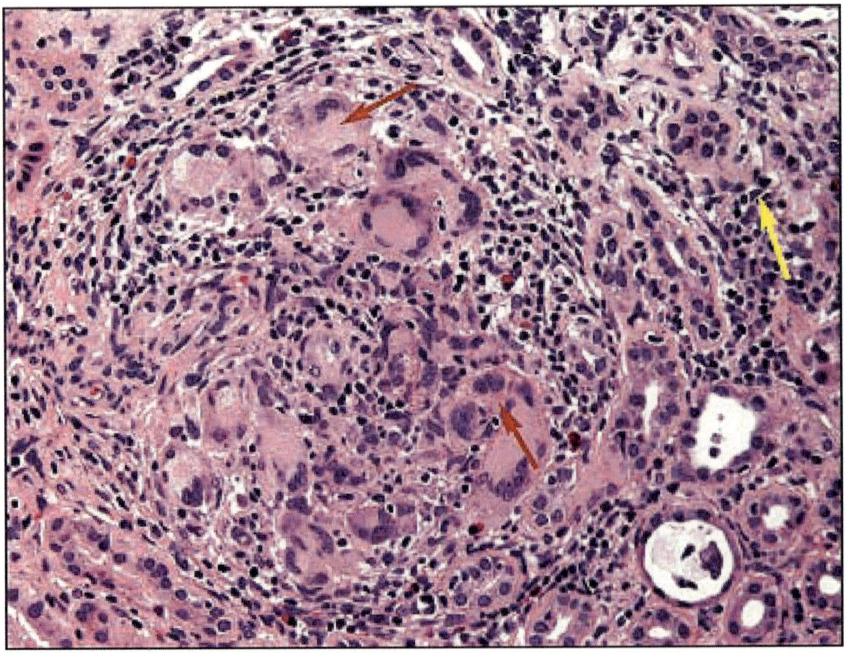

Figure 1.
Renal biopsy on light micrography shows noncaseating granulomata (red arrows) and patchy interstitial infiltrate (yellow arrow), with giant cells, inflammation, and moderate tubular atrophy and interstitial fibrosis.

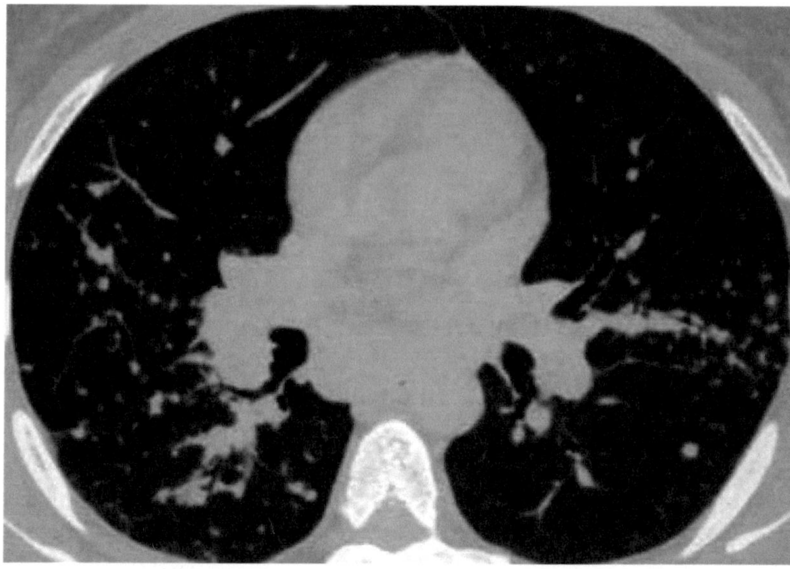

Figure 2.
A CT scan of the chest.

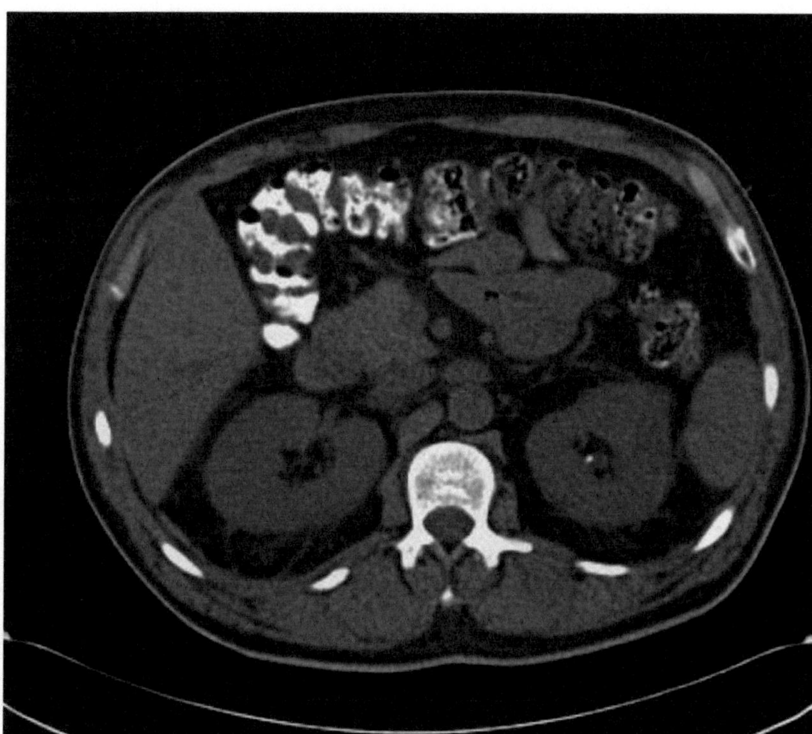

Figure 3.
A CT scan of the abdomen and pelvis.

4. Discussion

Histological findings in GIN may help to define the etiologic causes of granuloma. In sarcoidosis granulomatous inflammation is usually non-necrotizing, in contrast to those associated with antineutrophil cytoplasmic antibody (ANCA)-positive diseases such as granulomatosis with polyangiitis and infections such as tuberculosis [46]. Giant cells and granulomas also vary in number and can give some additional information but there is no clear pattern for a specific diagnosis [13, 48]. Bijol *et al.* reported that abundant granulomata are observed in GIN associated with sarcoidosis but are fewer in number when drugs are involved [38]. Moreover, the granulomas of sarcoidosis are described as 'naked' (i.e., without a rim of lymphocytes) [13] while abundant neutrophils and eosinophils, with ill-formed granulomas in a diffuse distribution, point again towards a drug-induced etiology [38]. Advanced sarcoidosis affecting the kidneys is characterized by marked interstitial fibrosis although the literature shows that many different causes of GIN associate various degrees of fibrosis. The presence of eosinophils was not helpful in diagnosing drug related pathology [13]. Immunofluorescence and electron microscopy are also not very helpful [46].

Granulomatous interstitial nephritis related to pyelonephritis or systemic infection has been noted to have an intense inflammatory infiltrate with lymphocytes, neutrophils and plasma cells, micro- abscess formation, white cell casts with or without papillary necrosis and vessel thrombosis and infarction. The number of macrophages, T and B cells are similar to those seen in GIN from other causes with an increase only in the number of neutrophils [49]. Infections with mycobacterial or fungal pathogens are usually associated with necrotizing granulomatous inflammation. The finding of caseous necrosis is more suggestive of tuberculosis (although this can be seen in other infections) [50]. However, this was only seen in 18.7% of cases of tuberculosis-GIN in one series [51]. In some cases, the infective agent can be readily identified with special stains (periodic acid-Schiff, Masson Trichrome, Silver and Ziehl-Nielsen or Auramine) [37, 38]. However, in certain cases, necrosis is absent, and granulomas may be poorly formed, therefore a high index of suspicion is needed.

Renal biopsies should be examined for possible etiologies of GIN especially microorganisms (acid fast bacili, fungi or viral inclusions) and some cases may require polymerase chain reaction (PCR) testing to support the diagnosis. Culture of fungi and mycobacteria is highly specific, but the result is often too delayed to be clinically meaningful at the time of the biopsy. Sometimes serologis tests like anti-Histoplasma antibodies may be helpful but one must keep in mind that early in the cpurse of the disease or in cases of immunocompromised patients the tests can have false-negative results [52]. Serum or urine detection of fungal antigens allows for a faster diagnosis but unfortunately the sensitivities vary [52]. A newer point-of-care test (XPert MTB/Rif) has been developed for detection of tuberculosis, but this has yet to be studied in histological specimens.

The diagnosis is even more difficult for the immunosuppressed patient as is shown in a recent study of HIV infected subjects [53]. In this population and in renal transplant recipients' infection is the leading cause of GIN. Tuberculosis is not only more frequent among the immunosuppressed, but immunosuppression may also alter the clinical picture and thereby obscure the diagnosis. An even more difficult situation appears in cases with the need to differentiate the acute interstitial nephritis in graft rejection from tubulitis of interstitial nephritis.

Oxalosis represents another etiology of GIN and renal biopsieis should be examined closely for crystals. Granulomas in the vicinity of vessels must be distinguished from vasculitis with granulomatous inflammation as seen in granulomatosis with polyangiitis. Fortunately both oxalosis and ANCA vasculitis are accompanied by other signs and symptoms which will aid in making the final and correct diagnosis. Finally, tubulorrhexis in acute tubular necrosis can be associated with granulomatous inflammation and must be distinguished from true GIN.

In our patient the initial differential diagnosis of hypercalcemia included many conditions. Hyperparathyroidism, malignancy (multiple myeloma, lymphoma, PTHrp associated malignancy and metastatic bone disease), infections (tuberculosis), sarcoid and vitamin D intoxication were all considered. Laboratory assessment narrowed the differential with an appropriately suppressed PTH and a low 25-hydroxyvitamin D level. The absence of lythic or blastic bone lesions made malignancy less likely. The elevated ACE level made sarcoid a strong possibility, and lymphomas was not readily considered as it can induce increased production of 1,25-D. Intrinsic renal disease was high on the differential rather than renal failure from nephrocalcinosis based on the following reasons: (1) while the hypercalcemia was slowly improving with intravenous hydration, the serum creatinine did not improve (2) the CT of the abdomen and pelvis showed a 3 mm non obstructing left renal calculus with normal size kidneys and no nephrocalcinosis. Moreover, the renal biopsy was required for definitive diagnosis.

5. Conclusion

Sarcoidosis, a multi-organ inflammatory disease that can also affect the kidney, should be considered as a potential diagnosis in any patient with hypercalcaemia and acute kidney injury. A renal biopsy will then have to be performed if other obvious causes such as myeloma, carcinoma with secondary metastases and primary hyperparathyroidism have been excluded. Acute kidney injury as the initial presentation of sarcoidosis is a rare entity. In some cases a number of patients with sarcoidosis have no extra renal manifestations of the disease upon presentation. Thus, all patients who have granulomatous interstitial nephritis detected on biopsy should have a chest radiograph, pulmonary function tests, and, if these are nondiagnostic, a high-resolution chest computed tomography (CT) scan should be performed to evaluate for pulmonary sarcoidosis.

Acute kidney injury without an "apparent" cause or resolution is an indication for an immediate renal biopsy to prevent further renal deterioration and allow for immediate treatment. Although usually sarcoidosis presents with more than one sign or symptom sometimes it may solely present as acute kidney injury. This type of sarcoidosis is a steroid-responsive disease and it is mandatory that a rapid diagnosis should be made and treatment should start as soon as possible in order to revent irreversible kidney damage.

Conflict of interest

The author declares no conflict of interest.

Author details

Marilena Stoian[1,2]

1 “Carol Davila” University of Medicine and Pharmacy, Bucharest, Romania

2 “Dr Ion Cantacuzino” Clinical Hospital, Bucharest, Romania

*Address all correspondence to: marilenastoian@yahoo.com

References

[1] Rossi G, Cavazza A, Colby TV. Pathology of sarcoidosis. Clinical Reviews in Allergy and Immunology. 2015;**49**:36

[2] Sakthivel P, Bruder D. Mechanism of granuloma formation in sarcoidosis. Current Opinion in Hematology. 2017;**24**:59

[3] Eberhardt C, Thillai M, Parker R, et al. Proteomic analysis of Kveim reagent identifies targets of cellular immunity in sarcoidosis. PLoS One. 2017;**12**:e0170285

[4] Grunewald J, Kaiser Y, Ostadkarampour M, et al. T-cell receptor-HLA-DRB1 associations suggest specific antigens in pulmonary sarcoidosis. The European Respiratory Journal. 2016;**47**:898

[5] Gorsane I, Zammouri A, Hajji M, et al. Renal involvement in sarcoidosis: Prognostic and predictive factors. Néphrologie & Thérapeutique. 2022;**18**:52

[6] Bergner R, Hoffmann M, Waldherr R, Uppenkamp M. Frequency of kidney disease in chronic sarcoidosis. Sarcoidosis, Vasculitis, and Diffuse Lung Diseases. 2003;**20**:126

[7] Lhote R, Annesi-Maesano I, Nunes H, et al. Clinical phenotypes of extrapulmonary sarcoidosis: An analysis of a French, multi-ethnic, multicentre cohort. The European Respiratory Journal. 2021;**57**

[8] Baughman RP, Teirstein AS, Judson MA, et al. Clinical characteristics of patients in case control study of sarcoidosis. American Journal of Respiratory and Critical Care Medicine. 2001;**164**:1885

[9] Schupp JC, Freitag-Wolf S, Bargagli E, et al. Phenotypes of organ involvement in sarcoidosis. The European Respiratory Journal. 2018;**51**

[10] Berliner AR, Haas M, Choi MJ. Sarcoidosis: The nephrologist's perspective. American Journal of Kidney Diseases. 2006;**48**:856

[11] Muther RS, McCarron DA, Bennett WM. Renal manifestations of sarcoidosis. Archives of Internal Medicine. 1981;**141**:643

[12] Rizzato G. Sarcoidosis in Italy. Sarcoidosis. 1992;**9**(Suppl. 1):145

[13] Joss N, Morris S, Young B, Geddes C. Granulomatous interstitial nephritis. Clinical Journal of the American Society of Nephrology. 2007;**2**:222-230

[14] Bergner R, Löffler C. Renal sarcoidosis: Approach to diagnosis and management. Current Opinion in Pulmonary Medicine. 2018;**24**:513

[15] Godin M, Fillastre JP, Ducastelle T, et al. Sarcoidosis. Retroperitoneal fibrosis, renal arterial involvement, and unilateral focal glomerulosclerosis. Archives of Internal Medicine. 1980;**140**:1240

[16] Gross KR, Malleson PN, Culham G, et al. Vasculopathy with renal artery stenosis in a child with sarcoidosis. The Journal of Pediatrics. 1986;**108**:724

[17] Mahévas M, Lescure FX, Boffa J-J, et al. Renal sarcoidosis: Clinical, laboratory, and histologic presentation and outcome in 47 patients. Medicine. 2009;**88**(2):98-106

[18] Aouizerate J, Matignon M, Kamar N, et al. Renal transplantation in patients

with sarcoidosis: A French multicenter study. Clinical Journal of the American Society of Nephrology. 2010;**5**:2101

[19] Mann DM, Fyfe B, Osband AJ, et al. Sarcoidosis within a renal allograft: A case report and review of the literature. Transplantation Proceedings. 2013;**45**:838

[20] Sharma OP. Vitamin D, calcium, and sarcoidosis. Chest. 1996;**109**(2):535-539

[21] Manjunath V, Moeckel G, Dahl NK. Acute kidney injury in a patient with sarcoidosis: Hypercalciuria and hypercalcemia leading to calcium phosphate deposition. Clinical Nephrology. 2013;**80**(2):151-155

[22] Gardner DG. Hypercalcemia and sarcoidosis—Another piece of the puzzle falls into place. American Journal of Medicine. 2001;**110**(9):736-737

[23] Reichel H, Koeffler HP, Barbers R, Norman AW. Regulation of 1,25-dihydroxyvitamin D_3 production by cultured alveolar macrophages from normal human donors and from patients with pulmonary sarcoidosis. The Journal of Clinical Endocrinology & Metabolism. 1987;**65**(6):1201-1209

[24] Adams JS, Sharma OP, Gacad MA, Singer FR. Metabolism of 25-hydroxyvitamin D3 by cultured pulmonary alveolar macrophages in sarcoidosis. The Journal of Clinical Investigation. 1983;**72**(5):1856-1860

[25] Mason RS, Frankel T, Chan YL, Lissner D, Posen S. Vitamin D conversion by sarcoid lymph node homogenate. Annals of Internal Medicine. 1984;**100**(1):59-61

[26] Insogna KL, Dreyer BE, Mitnick M, et al. Enhanced production rate of 1,25-dihydroxyvitamin D in sarcoidosis. The Journal of Clinical Endocrinology and Metabolism. 1988;**66**:72

[27] Inui N, Murayama A, Sasaki S, et al. Correlation between 25-hydroxyvitamin D3 1 alpha-hydroxylase gene expression in alveolar macrophages and the activity of sarcoidosis. The American Journal of Medicine. 2001;**110**:687

[28] Zeimer HJ, Greenaway TM, Slavin J, et al. Parathyroid-hormone-related protein in sarcoidosis. The American Journal of Pathology. 1998;**152**:17

[29] Iannuzzi MC, Rybicki BA, Teirstein AS. Sarcoidosis. The New England Journal of Medicine. 2007;**357**(21):2153-2165

[30] Basile JN, Liel Y, Shary J, Bell NH. Increased calcium intake does not suppress circulating 1,25-dihydroxyvitamin D in normocalcemic patients with sarcoidosis. The Journal of Clinical Investigation. 1993;**91**:1396

[31] Levi M, Peterson L, Berl T. Mechanism of concentrating defect in hypercalcemia. Role of polydipsia and prostaglandins. Kidney International. 1983;**23**:489

[32] Reid JD, Andersen ME. Calcium oxalate in sarcoid granulomas. With particular reference to the small ovoid body and a note on the finding of dolomite. American Journal of Clinical Pathology. 1988;**90**(5):545-558

[33] Komatsuda A, Wakui H, Ohtani H, et al. Amyloid A-type renal amyloidosis in a patient with sarcoidosis: Report of a case and review of the literature. Clinical Nephrology. 2003;**60**:284

[34] Mariano RT, Sussman SK. Sarcoidosis of the ureter. AJR. American Journal of Roentgenology. 1998;**171**:1431

[35] Casella FJ, Allon M. The kidney in sarcoidosis. Journal of American Society Nephrology. 1993;**3**:1555-1562

[36] O'Riordan E, Willert RP, Reeve R, Kalra PA, O'Donoghue DJ, Foley RN, et al. Isolated sarcoid granulomatous interstitial nephritis: Review of five cases at one center. Clinical Nephrology. 2001;**55**:297-302

[37] Naidu GD, Ram R, Swarnalatha G, et al. Granulomatous interstitial nephritis: Our experience of 14 patients. Indian Journal of Nephrology. 2013;**23**:415-418

[38] Bijol V, Mendez GP, Nosé V, Rennke HG. Granulomatous interstitial nephritis: A clinicopathologic study of 46 cases from a single institution. International Journal of Surgical Pathology. 2006;**14**:57-63

[39] Javaud N, Belenfant X, Stirnemann J, Laederich J, Ziol M, Callard P, et al. Renal granulomatoses: A retrospective study of 40 cases and review of the literature. Medicine. 2007;**86**:170-180

[40] Javaud N, Belenfant X, Stirnemann J, et al. Renal granulomatoses: A retrospective study of 40 cases and review of the literature. Medicine (Baltimore). 2007;**86**:170-180

[41] Balafa O, Liapis G, Duni A, Xiromeriti S, Kalaitzidis R, Elisaf M. An unusual case of acute kidney injury – Idiopathic granulomatous tubulointerstitial nephritis. Clinical Nephrology. 2015;**84**:247-250

[42] Mignon F, Mery JP, Mougenot B, et al. Granulomatous interstitial nephritis. Advances in Nephrology from the Necker Hospital. 1984;**13**:219-245

[43] Ikeda A, Nagai S, Kitaichi M, et al. Sarcoidosis with granulomatous interstitial nephritis: Report of three cases. Internal Medicine. 2001;**40**:241-245

[44] Ramakrishnan L. Revisiting the role of the granuloma in tuberculosis. Nature Reviews. Immunology. 2012;**12**:352-366

[45] Rosen Y. Pathology of sarcoidosis. Seminars in Respiratory and Critical Care Medicine. 2007;**28**:36-52

[46] Broos CE, van Nimwegen M, Hoogsteden HC, et al. Granuloma formation in pulmonary sarcoidosis. Frontiers in Immunology. 2013;**4**:437

[47] Chopra A, Brasher P, Chaudhry H, et al. Proteinuria in sarcoidosis: Prevalence and risk factors in a consecutive outpatient cohort. Sarcoidosis, Vasculitis, and Diffuse Lung Diseases. 2017;**34**:142

[48] Shah S, Carter-Monroe N, Atta MG. Granulomatous interstitial nephritis. Clinical Kidney Journal. 2015;**8**:516-523

[49] Viero RM, Cavallo T. Granulomatous interstitial nephritis. Human Pathology. 1995;**26**:1347-1353

[50] Chung S, Park CW, Chung HW, et al. Acute renal failure presenting as a granulomatous interstitial nephritis due to cryptococcal infection. Kidney International. 2009;**76**:453-458

[51] Chapagain A, Dobbie H, Sheaff M, et al. Presentation, diagnosis, and treatment outcome of tuberculous-mediated tubulointerstitial nephritis. Kidney International. 2011;**79**:671-677

[52] Qian Q, Humayun H, Humayun Y, et al. Granulomatous interstitial nephritis associated with disseminated histoplasmosis in an immunocompetent patient. American Journal of Kidney Diseases. 2011;**58**:1018-1102

[53] Nel D. A Retrospective Review of Granulomatous Interstitial Nephritis (GIN) amongst HIV-Infected Patients at Groote Schuur Hospital Cape Town. Cape Town: Faculty of Health Sciences, University of Cape Town; 2014

Chapter 7

Sarcoidosis of the Breast

Cedric Pluguez-Turull, Cinthia Del Toro and Youley Tjendra

Abstract

The clinical manifestation of breast sarcoidosis accounts for <1% of cases of sarcoidosis and typically presents in the setting of already documented systemic involvement. Within the breast, sarcoidosis can often present as a firm palpable mass in young or middle-aged women. On mammography, imaging findings range from small, well-defined round masses to irregular, spiculated masses. Ultrasound most commonly demonstrates an ill-defined hypoechoic mass. As a result, breast sarcoidosis can mimic benign and malignant pathologies such as fat necrosis, fibroadenoma or breast cancer. This variability in imaging appearance represents a diagnostic challenge often culminating in image-guided or surgical biopsy and histological analysis to establish a definitive diagnosis. Ultimately, while breast involvement is uncommon, it accentuates the diverse clinical manifestations of sarcoidosis, which may be clinically suspected and must be adequately evaluated to exclude more significant pathologies.

Keywords: breast, sarcoidosis, granulomas, mammography, ultrasound, MRI, granulomatous, inflammation, mastitis, autoimmune

1. Introduction

Sarcoidosis is a chronic multisystemic disease characterized by the formation of granulomas in various organs as a consequence of an antigen-driven inflammatory response of unknown etiology [1]. These noncaseating granulomatous lesions most commonly affect the lungs and intrathoracic lymph nodes, but can also be found in the skin, eyes, liver, and less frequently, the breasts. Breast sarcoidosis accounts for less than 1% of sarcoidosis cases and typically presents in the setting of widespread disease [2]. The complexity of the clinical presentation is a major factor in prolonging the time to diagnosis and contributing to the lack of or inappropriate treatment [3]. The criteria for the diagnosis of sarcoidosis are largely subjective and have yet to be standardized. This makes way for the misdiagnosis of sarcoidosis with other granulomatous diseases because of the similarity and overlap of clinical, radiographic, and histological features, which poses a diagnostic dilemma [4].

Mammography and ultrasonography are the first-line imaging modalities most utilized in breast imaging, while magnetic resonance imaging (MRI) is used more secondarily as a problem-solving tool or after a diagnosis has been made for treatment planning. Imaging in breast sarcoidosis is usually followed by histological analysis of the symptomatic or incidentally encountered breast mass, regardless of the level of suspicion of sarcoidosis, unless the main differential diagnoses include benign and probably benign findings for which short–interval follow up is opted to document long term stability. The presence of non-necrotizing granulomas suggests a diagnosis of breast sarcoidosis, particularly if supporting clinical factors and past medical history are present. Once the diagnosis is established, corticosteroid therapy may be considered as a first-line treatment [1].

The purpose of this chapter is to explore the clinical, radiological, and histopathological presentation of breast sarcoidosis, focusing on conventional imaging methods while addressing the challenges associated with an accurate and timely diagnosis.

2. Epidemiology and demographics

Identifying risk factors, and patterns in the distribution and occurrence of sarcoidosis can aid our understanding of the disease and help build a framework geared towards disease prevention. Epidemiologic studies have shown the highest incidence and prevalence rates to be in African American patients and in patients in the Nordic region. The lowest incidence and prevalence rates were seen in Hispanic and Asian patients [5]. Sarcoidosis generally affects 20 to 40-year-old individuals with a higher prevalence in women (1.3%) than in men (1%). African American women have the highest disease prevalence [6]. However, the true incidence and prevalence of sarcoidosis remains undetermined because of the fact that many patients are asymptomatic [7].

Variations in the age and presentation between men and women have been reported in the literature but the data remains inconsistent. One of the most consistent findings across multiple studies is the reduced risk of sarcoidosis in individuals who smoke compared to individuals who do not smoke [5].

Potential risk factors of sarcoidosis include obesity, having a first degree relative with sarcoidosis, and having a history of infection. A diagnosis of sarcoidosis in more than one family member suggests that genetics holds a potential role in the disease process [1, 8]. Conversely, several studies have reported sarcoidosis as a risk factor for malignancy [5].

3. Clinical presentation

Breast sarcoidosis is most often seen in the setting of systemic disease, but it can also be the primary manifestation of sarcoidosis [7]. The workup can ensue after abnormal findings are detected on either a screening mammography, a screening breast ultrasound, or as a result of an incidental finding on chest imaging. These patients typically present without any complaints or breast masses [2, 3, 9]. Symptomatic patients, on the other hand, usually present because of a self-detected breast mass [10]. In general, clinical manifestations of breast sarcoidosis can be unilateral or bilateral and may include: palpable mass, breast tenderness, lymphadenopathy, nipple changes, and skin abnormalities [6, 7, 11].

In most breast sarcoidosis cases, the physical exam on initial presentation reveals a single firm, mobile, and non-tender mass. Prior pooled studies have described mass diameter ranges from 0.25 to 5 cm in size. Enlarged ipsilateral axillary lymph nodes is also fairly common and is well within the purview of a typical breast focused clinical and imaging examination. Fixed or painful lesions are less common clinical manifestations. When present, skin findings can include skin retraction, dimpling, or *peau d'orange* appearance. Interestingly, one reported case of breast sarcoidosis erythematous skin changes of the breast with brown pigmentation, flaky skin, and palpable induration on exam was described. Nipple retraction and discharge have been rarely reported [2, 10, 11].

Although more commonly observed in females, breast sarcoidosis can also affect male patients. In searching the literature, only one case report involving male breast tissue was found. An African American man with an established diagnosis of lung sarcoidosis presented with bilateral breast tenderness and palpable nodules determined to be sarcoidosis involving the breast tissue after biopsy [6].

Given the heterogeneity of this clinical presentation, the differential diagnosis often includes benign and malignant disease processes such as a fibroadenoma, mastitis, idiopathic granulomatous mastitis, and certainly breast cancer. While malignancy is the most important diagnosis to rule out in a patient presenting with a symptomatic breast finding, it is important to consider common benign etiologies to manage them accordingly. For a palpable tender breast mass of acute onset, a mastitis may be considered, and management may begin with the least invasive intervention, such as starting with antibiotics and a follow-up ultrasound [1]. An elevated serum level of angiotensin-converting enzyme (ACE) is a strong indicator of sarcoidosis but has poor specificity and renders it an unreliable biomarker for diagnostic purposes. As a result, histologic evidence of sarcoidosis in breast tissue is most often necessary for diagnosis [11, 12].

4. Pathology

Sarcoidosis is a multisystemic disease of unknown etiology characterized by non-necrotizing granulomas. The lymphatic system is one of the most commonly affected sites [13–16]. Rarely, the breast may be affected by systemic sarcoidosis and is usually, but not exclusively, detected after the diagnosis has been established [17–19].

Given the lack of specific diagnostic biomarkers, histologic evidence of a granuloma is not uncommonly required to establish an accurate diagnosis. Granulomas are composed of tightly clustered epithelioid histiocytes, occasional multinucleated giant cells of Langhans type, and lymphocytes. An outer layer of loosely organized lymphocytes and dendritic cells is often observed. A concentric arrangement of epithelioid histiocytes around a large, multinucleated giant cell of the Langhans can also be identified. Asteroid bodies, cytoskeleton filaments, and lipoproteins located within the cytoplasm of giant cells, or Schaumann bodies, basophilic to black, concentrically laminated structures, may be seen. Necrosis is usually absent throughout the lesion. An example of systemic sarcoidosis involving the axillary lymph node and primary breast sarcoidosis of the right breast is shown in **Figures 1** and **2**, respectively.

The differential diagnoses of granulomatous inflammation involving the axillary lymph node or breast include infectious granulomatosis (i.e., tuberculosis, mycobacterial infection), inflammatory diseases with granulomatous reaction, drug-induced sarcoid-like reactions, or tumor-associated sarcoid-like reactions (i.e., lymphomas, carcinomas) [20].

5. Imaging

Breast sarcoidosis is a rare manifestation of systemic sarcoidosis, and its imaging features are important for diagnosis and appropriate management. The imaging

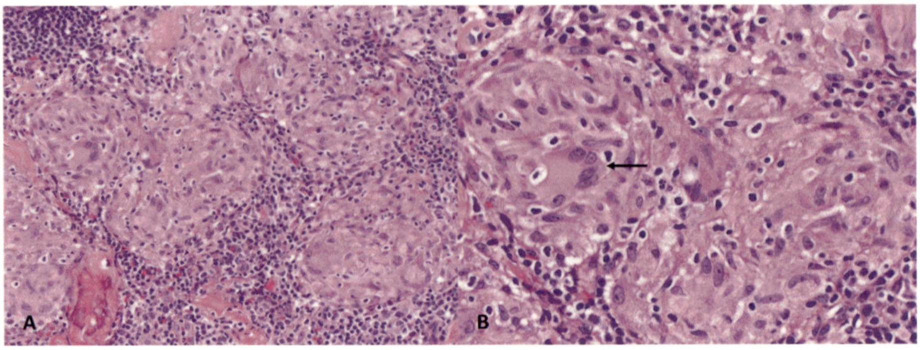

Figure 1.
Axillary lymph node involvement by systemic sarcoidosis. A–B. Histologic sections show tightly clustered epithelioid histiocytes with multinucleated giant cells of Langhans type (→). Intervening and scattered lymphocytes are small and without atypia. (Hematoxylin and Eosin [H&E], A. 20×, B. 40×).

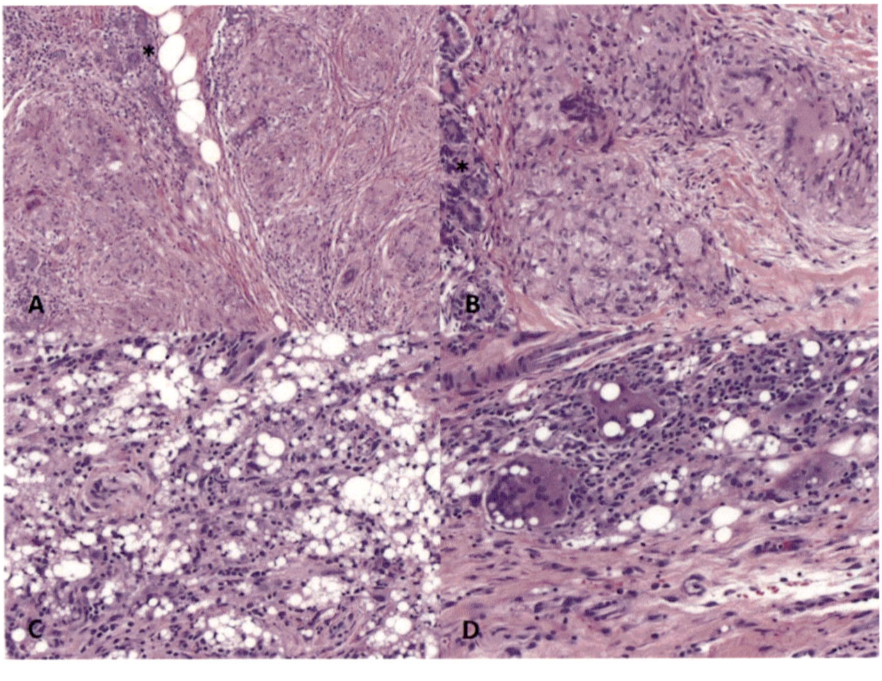

Figure 2.
Breast sarcoidosis involving the right upper-inner quadrant of a 47-year-old female. A–B. Sections show mammary parenchyma with epithelioid granulomas forming nodules with multinucleated Langhans giant cells among ducts and lobules (*). Necrosis or central microabscesses are not identified (Hematoxylin and Eosin [H&E], A. 10×, B. 20×). C-D. The differential diagnosis includes granulomatous reaction to foreign material (silicone; H&E, C. 10×, D. 20×).

characteristics of breast sarcoidosis have been studied across various modalities, and available literature provides valuable insights into this uncommon condition.

Mammography plays a crucial role in the initial evaluation of breast sarcoidosis. Reis et al. (2019) conducted a study involving 12 patients with breast sarcoidosis, where mammographic findings revealed ill-defined masses with dense, irregular margins in 83% of cases. These masses exhibited asymmetric density or focal architectural distortion which has been described as a high density mass with spiculated margins [2, 21]. Calcifications were relatively uncommon, observed in only 17% of the patients, and when present, they tended to be fine and punctate. However, it is important to note that mammographic features of breast sarcoidosis are non-specific and can overlap with other benign or malignant breast conditions, necessitating histopathological confirmation for accurate diagnosis [2].

Ultrasound is another valuable imaging modality for evaluating breast sarcoidosis. A study by Huang et al. (2010) included 14 patients with biopsy-proven breast sarcoidosis where findings demonstrated hypoechoic masses with irregular margins in 71% of the cases. Furthermore, posterior acoustic shadowing, suggesting a dense or solid nature of the masses, was observed in 79% of patients. Sarcoidosis can be seen as a solitary irregular mass, but can also be seen as multiple masses [21, 22]. In some cases, diffuse hypoechoic parenchymal changes without distinct masses have been documented. The use of a linear high frequency probe with high-resolution probe can help evaluate better the characteristic irregular margins with spiculations, and heterogenous echotexture of the classic sarcoidosis mass finding [23]. However, similar to mammography, ultrasonographic features of breast sarcoidosis are non-specific and may mimic other breast pathologies. Therefore, biopsy remains necessary for definitive diagnosis [24].

Magnetic Resonance Imaging (MRI) is an additional tool for evaluation of breast sarcoidosis with functional imaging features emphasizing degree of vascularity and molecular composition. In a study by Huang et al. (2010), MRI findings of 12 patients with breast sarcoidosis revealed most masses demonstrated low to intermediate signal intensity on T1-weighted images and high signal intensity on T2-weighted images. After gadolinium-based contrast administration, these masses demonstrated heterogeneous mass enhancement. However, MRI features also resemble other inflammatory or neoplastic breast conditions. Histopathological confirmation through biopsy remains necessary for definitive diagnosis [24].

Fluorine 18 fluorodeoxyglucose (FDG) positron emission tomography (PET)-computed tomography (CT) is used to detect metabolically active lesions typically in the setting of malignancy. The imaging features and patterns of sarcoidosis on FDG PET/CT varies and can mimic lymphatic cancer and metastatic disease because of the common finding of intrathoracic lymphadenopathy [25]. In general, enlarged lymph nodes with increased FDG uptake are revealed on axial plain CT, PET, and PET-CT fusion images [26, 27]. Zivin et al. (2014) report a case of a patient with known breast cancer and histologically confirmed sarcoidosis, which was initially thought to be metastatic cancer. The presence of concurrent sarcoidosis was detected on FDG PET/CT as hypermetabolic mediastinal and hilar lymph nodes in a "butterfly" distribution pattern [28]. Sarcoidosis and breast cancer have been documented to occur simultaneously, which given the relative rarity of the disease, diagnosis can often be confounded by concomitant cancer [29].

Molecular breast imaging (MBI) provides functional information about breast sarcoidosis by using Tecnecium-99 sestamibi radiotracer. Cattaneo et al. (2012) reported a case series of four patients with breast sarcoidosis who underwent MBI. The MBI findings showed areas of increased radiotracer uptake corresponding to inflammatory granulomas in all cases. However, due to its limited anatomical detail, MBI should be used in conjunction with other imaging modalities to achieve an accurate diagnosis [30].

Contrast-enhanced mammography (CEM), which uses intravenous iodinated contrast agents, can enhance the visualization of breast lesions. Reis et al. (2021)

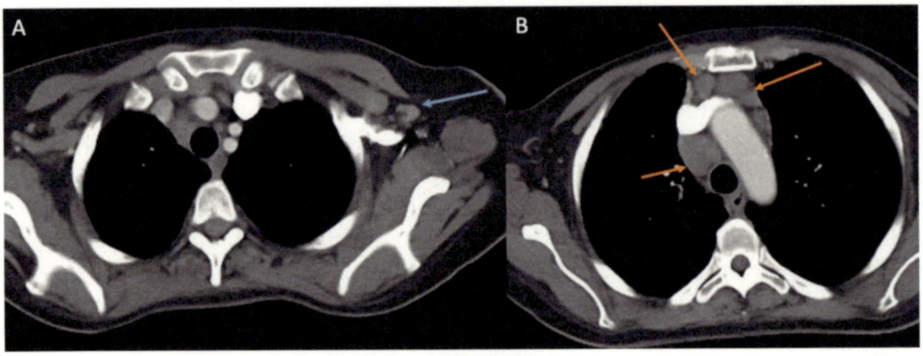

Figure 3.
Axial contrast enhanced chest CT in a patient with a known history of breast cancer. A. There is a prominent left axillary lymph node measuring 1.1 cm (blue arrow). B. Extensive multi station mediastinal adenopathy including a 2.3 cm right upper paratracheal lymph node, 2.6 cm subcarinal lymph node, 1.2 cm para-aortic node and 1.5 cm preaortic lymph node (orange arrows).

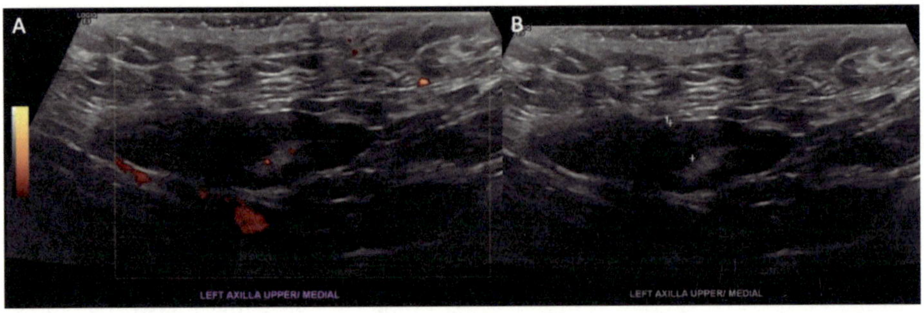

Figure 4.
Limited left axillary ultrasound. A. The Power Doppler technique showing hilar vascularity. B. An enlarged lymph node in the left axilla with cortical thickness of up to 0.5 cm.

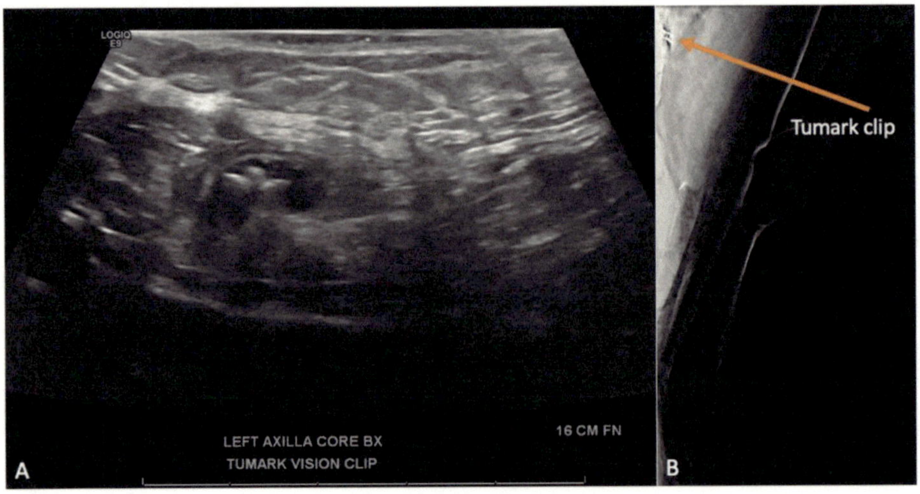

Figure 5.
Ultrasound guided core needle biopsy of enlarged left axillary lymph node. A. Several core needle biopsy passes performed followed by clip placement. B. Tumark clip shown on mammogram after biopsy.

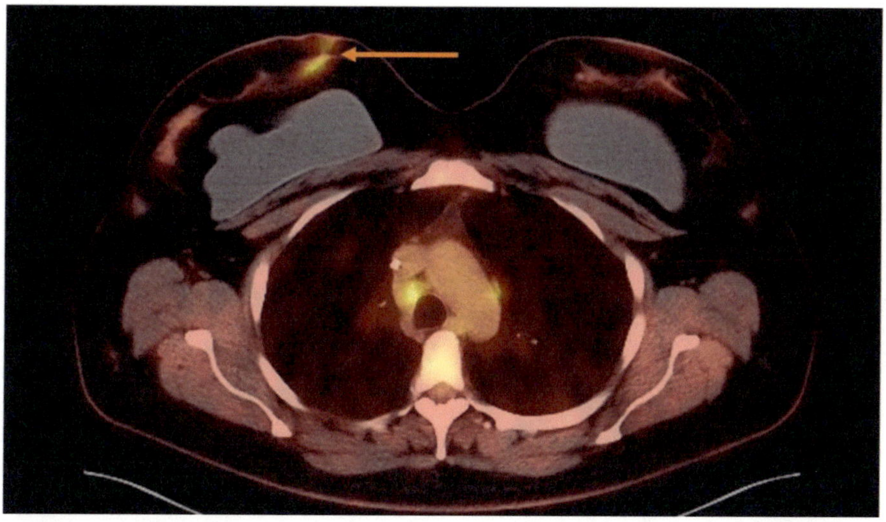

Figure 6.
Nuclear Medicine PET/CT Chest. FDG avid subcutaneous lesions noted in the upper inner right breast (orange arrow).

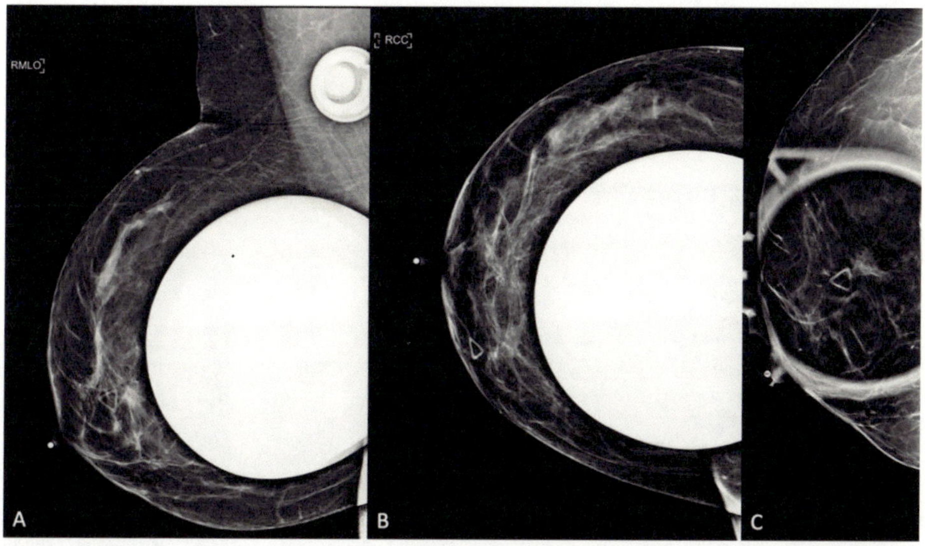

Figure 7.
Digital diagnostic cranial caudal and mediolateral oblique views of the right breast obtained with and without implant displacement. A. There is a 1.2 × 1.1 × 1.1 cm irregular, spiculated mass, superficial in location, with questionable spiculations extending to the overlying skin. B, C. An area of architectural distortion in the right outer breast, middle depth, 6 cm from nipple improves on additional spot compression views favoring tissue summation. 0.4 cm round circumscribed mass in the right retro-areolar breast. Focal asymmetry in the right upper outer breast, middle and posterior depths favoring tissue summation on tomosynthesis imaging.

studied 12 patients with breast sarcoidosis and reported that contrast-enhanced mammography revealed irregular masses with focal enhancement patterns in 67% of the cases [1]. See imaging examples in **Figures 3–9**.

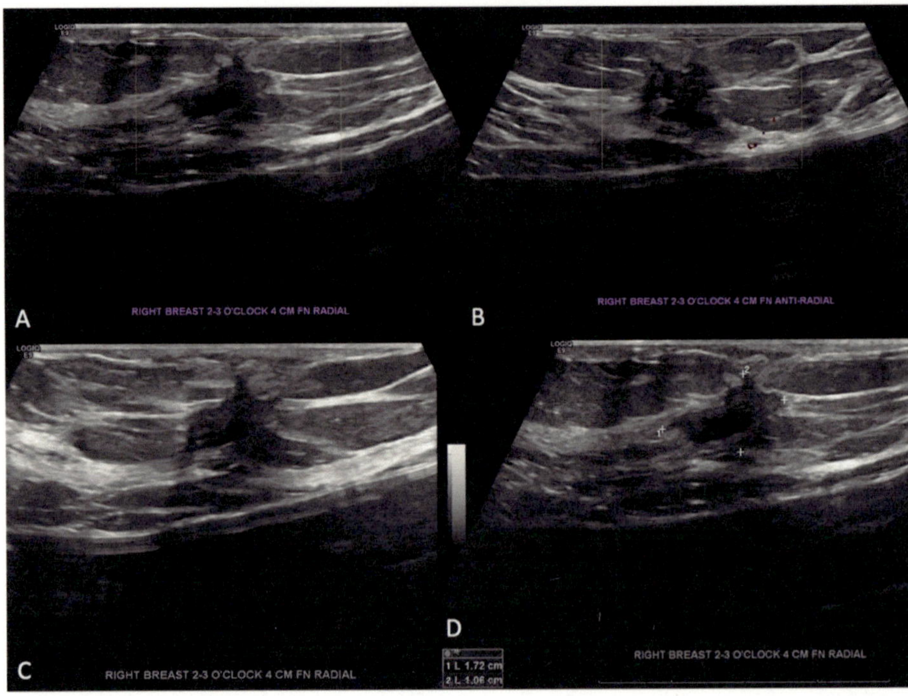

Figure 8.
Breast ultrasound. A-D 1.7 cm irregular mass correlates with PET CT FSG avid mass and mammogram finding under the palpable site and is deemed highly suspicious for breast malignancy – BIRADS 5.

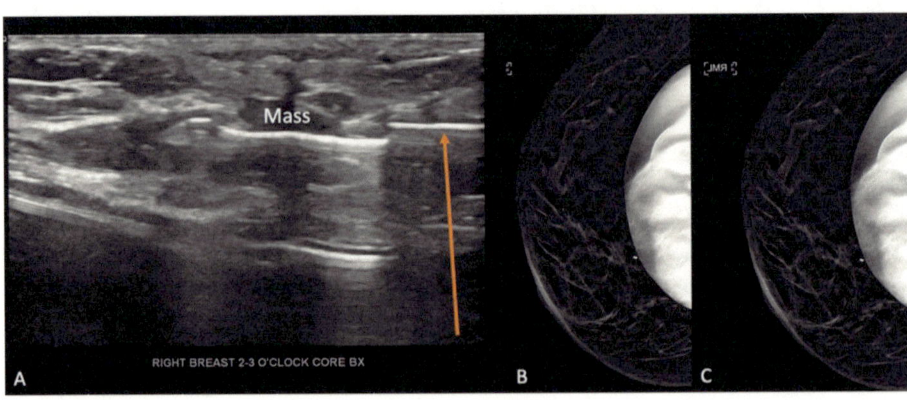

Figure 9.
Ultrasound-guided core needle biopsy of suspicious mass in right breast. A. Core needle visualized near mass during biopsy (orange arrow). B, C. Right cranial caudal and mediolateral oblique views on mammogram demonstrate that the biopsy clip corresponds to the abnormality on the mammogram which is under the triangle marker representing the palpable area of concern.

6. Management

Sarcoidosis of the breast is managed with the purpose of removing the granulomatous tissue. Treatment options include corticosteroids, surgery, or a combination of both along with close follow-up care [6]. Standard dose corticosteroid therapy is the treatment of choice for breast sarcoidosis and should be started as soon as possible. The dosage should be tapered gradually as well [11]. Some authors advise that the adverse effects associated with long-term steroid use should be weighed against the degree of diseased tissue and functional impairment when deciding whether to treat or not [31]. An immunosuppressive therapeutic regimen is not indicated in sarcoidosis localized to the breasts, which may be related to increased risk of skin cancers, non-Hodgkin lymphoma and infection while hospitalized [1, 5]. Surgical management is rarely implemented but can be considered in the setting of more severely symptomatic or larger disease extent [6]. Symptomatic patients can be monitored with clinical and breast imaging surveillance, usually breast ultrasound, at regular time intervals until there is complete resolution of symptoms and improvement or stability of breast finding is achieved [7].

Ultimately, multidisciplinary collaboration between the breast radiologist, the pathologist, and the primary care provider or other treating clinician is necessary to reach a prompt diagnosis, expedite management and optimize clinical outcomes.

7. Conclusion

In conclusion, breast sarcoidosis presents a diagnostic challenge due to its non-specific imaging features on various modalities. The studies conducted on small cohorts of patients have provided valuable insights into the imaging characteristics of breast sarcoidosis. Mammography, ultrasound, MRI, FDG PET/CT, MBI, and CEM may all reveal characteristic findings that can suggest breast sarcoidosis in the appropriate clinical context. However, histopathological examination remains essential for definitive diagnosis and appropriate management of this rare disease.

Author details

Cedric Pluguez-Turull[1*], Cinthia Del Toro[2] and Youley Tjendra[3]

1 Breast Imaging Section University of Miami Health System and Miller School of Medicine, Miami, United States

2 University of Miami Miller School of Medicine, Miami, United States

3 Pathology Department of University of Miami Health System and Miller School of Medicine, Miami, United States

*Address all correspondence to: cedricpluguez@miami.edu

References

[1] Reis J, Boavida J, Bahrami N, Lyngra M, Geitung JT. Breast sarcoidosis: Clinical features, imaging, and histological findings. The Breast Journal. 2021;**27**(1):44-47. DOI: 10.1111/tbj.14075

[2] Reis J, Boavida J, Lyngra M, Geitung JT. Radiological evaluation of primary breast sarcoidosis presenting as bilateral breast lesions. BMJ Case Report. 2019;**12**(7):e229591. Published 2019 Jul 27. DOI: 10.1136/bcr-2019-229591

[3] Jaguś D, Yafimtsau I, Mlosek RK, Jonczak L, Roszkowska-Purska K, Dobruch-Sobczak K. Sarcoidosis of the breasts – When should it be considered? A case report. Journal of Ultrasonic. 2022;**22**(89):136-139. Published 2022 Apr 27. DOI: 10.15557/JoU.2022.0022

[4] Judson MA. Granulomatous sarcoidosis mimics. Frontier in Medicine (Lausanne). 2021;**8**:680989. Published 2021 Jul 8. DOI: 10.3389/fmed.2021.680989

[5] Arkema EV, Cozier YC. Epidemiology of sarcoidosis: Current findings and future directions. Therapeutic Advance in Chronic Disease. 2018;**9**(11):227-240. Published 2018 Aug 24. DOI: 10.1177/2040622318790197

[6] Grove J, Meier C, Youssef B, Costello P. A rare case of sarcoidosis involving male breast tissue. Cureus. 2022;**14**(1):e21387. Published 2022 Jan 18. DOI: 10.7759/cureus.21387

[7] Rhazari M, Ramdani A, Gartini S, et al. Mammary sarcoidosis: A rare case report. Annals of Medical Surgery (Lond). 2022;**78**:103892. Published 2022 May 31. DOI: 10.1016/j.amsu.2022.103892

[8] Arkema EV, Cozier YC. Sarcoidosis epidemiology: Recent estimates of incidence, prevalence, and risk factors. Current Opinion in Pulmonary Medicine. 2020;**26**(5):527-534. DOI: 10.1097/MCP.0000000000000715

[9] Mason C, Yang R, Hamilton R, et al. Diagnosis of sarcoidosis from a biopsy of a dilated mammary duct. Proceedings (Baylor University Medical Center). 2017;**30**(2):197-199. DOI: 10.1080/08998280.2017.11929584

[10] Ojeda H, Sardi A, Totoonchie A. Sarcoidosis of the breast: implications for the general surgeon. The American Surgeon. 2000;**66**(12):1144-1148

[11] Zujić PV, Grebić D, Valenčić L. Chronic granulomatous inflammation of the breast as a first clinical manifestation of primary sarcoidosis. Breast Care (Basel). 2015;**10**(1):51-53. DOI: 10.1159/000370206

[12] Doan T, Nguyen NT, He J, Nguyen QD. Sarcoidosis presenting in breast imaging clinic with unilateral axillary lymphadenopathy. Cureus. 2021;**13**(2):e13245. Published 2021 Feb 9. DOI: 10.7759/cureus.13245

[13] Sikjær MG, Hilberg O, Ibsen R, Løkke A. Sarcoidosis: A nationwide registry-based study of incidence, prevalence and diagnostic work-up. Respiratory Medicine. 2021;**187**:106548. DOI: 10.1016/j.rmed.2021.106548

[14] Caplan A, Rosenbach M, Imadojemu S. Cutaneous sarcoidosis. Seminars in Respiratory and Critical Care Medicine. 2020;**41**(5):689-699. DOI: 10.1055/s-0040-1713130

[15] Mañá J, Rubio-Rivas M, Villalba N, et al. Multidisciplinary approach and long-term follow-up in a series of 640

consecutive patients with sarcoidosis: Cohort study of a 40-year clinical experience at a tertiary referral center in Barcelona, Spain. Medicine (Baltimore). 2017;**96**(29):e7595. DOI: 10.1097/MD.0000000000007595

[16] Bodaghi B, Touitou V, Fardeau C, Chapelon C, LeHoang P. Ocular sarcoidosis. Presse Médicale. 2012;**41** (6 Pt. 2):e349-e354. DOI: 10.1016/j.lpm.2012.04.004

[17] Takahashi R, Shibuya Y, Shijubo N, Asaishi K, Abe S. Mammary involvement in a patient with sarcoidosis. Internal Medicine. 2001;**40**(8):769-771. DOI: 10.2169/internalmedicine.40.769

[18] Fiorucci F, Conti V, Lucantoni G, et al. Sarcoidosis of the breast: A rare case report and a review. European Review for Medical and Pharmacological Sciences. 2006;**10**(2):47-50

[19] Gansler TS, Wheeler JE. Mammary sarcoidosis. Two cases and literature review. Archives of Pathology & Laboratory Medicine. 1984;**108**(8):673-675

[20] El Jammal T, Jamilloux Y, Gerfaud-Valentin M, Valeyre D, Sève P. Refractory sarcoidosis: A review. Therapeutics and Clinical Risk Management. 2020;**16**:323-345. Published 2020 Apr 17. DOI: 10.2147/TCRM.S192922

[21] Naeem M, Zulfiqar M, Ballard DH, et al. "The unusual suspects"-Mammographic, sonographic, and histopathologic appearance of atypical breast masses. Clinical Imaging. 2020;**66**:111-120. DOI: 10.1016/j.clinimag.2020.04.039

[22] Ishimaru K, Isomoto I, Okimoto T, Itoyanagi A, Uetani M. Sarcoidosis of the breast. European Radiology. 2002;**12**(Suppl. 3):S105-S108. DOI: 10.1007/s00330-002-1627-4

[23] Kenzel PP, Hadijuana J, Hosten N, et al. Boeck sarcoidosis of the breast: mammographic, ultrasound, and MR findings. Journal of Computer Assisted Tomography. 1997;**21**(3):439-441. DOI: 10.1097/00004728-199705000-00018

[24] Huang C, Chang YC, Huang WY, et al. Breast sarcoidosis: Mammographic, sonographic, and MRI findings. Journal of Clinical Ultrasound. 2010;**38**(5):262-266. DOI: 10.1002/jcu.20689

[25] Prabhakar HB, Rabinowitz CB, Gibbons FK, O'Donnell WJ, Shepard JA, Aquino SL. Imaging features of sarcoidosis on MDCT, FDG PET, and PET/CT. AJR. American Journal of Roentgenology. 2008;**190**(3 Suppl):S1-S6. DOI: 10.2214/AJR.07.7001

[26] Li YJ, Zhang Y, Gao S, Bai RJ. Cervical and axillary lymph node sarcoidosis misdiagnosed as lymphoma on F-18 FDG PET-CT. Clinical Nuclear Medicine. 2007;**32**(3):262-264. DOI: 10.1097/01.rlu.0000255268.64309.8e

[27] Akaike G, Itani M, Shah H, et al. PET/CT in the diagnosis and workup of sarcoidosis: Focus on atypical manifestations. Radiographics. 2018;**38**(5):1536-1549. DOI: 10.1148/rg.2018180053

[28] Zivin S, David O, Lu Y. Sarcoidosis mimicking metastatic breast cancer on FDG PET/CT. Internal Medicine. 2014;**53**(21):2555-2556. DOI: 10.2169/internalmedicine.53.3333

[29] Altınkaya M, Altınkaya N, Hazar B. Sarcoidosis mimicking metastatic breast cancer in a patient with early-stage breast cancer. Ulus Cerrahi Derg.

2015;**32**(1):71-74. Published 2015 Jul 6. DOI: 10.5152/UCD.2015.2989

[30] Cattaneo E, Lippolis PV, Gasparini E, et al. Breast sarcoidosis: Imaging features of a rare disease. AJR. American Journal of Roentgenology. 2012;**199**(1):W112-W116. DOI: 10.2214/AJR.11.7179

[31] Endlich JL, Souza JA, Osório CABT, Pinto CAL, Faria EP, Bitencourt AGV. Breast sarcoidosis as the first manifestation of the disease. The Breast Journal. 2020;**26**(3):543-544. DOI: 10.1111/tbj.13560

Chapter 8

Anti-Granulomatous Therapy for Pulmonary Sarcoidosis

Alicia K. Gerke

Abstract

Sarcoidosis is a systemic disease of granulomatous inflammation that predominately affects the lungs. The cause is unknown. Although over half of cases spontaneously resolve, a large proportion of patients require therapy for progressive symptoms or worsening organ function. Corticosteroids remain first-line therapy, but steroid-sparing medications should be considered in high-risk cases. In this chapter, we review types of therapies targeted to the granulomatous inflammatory pathway and their role in treatment of sarcoidosis. Because of the complex interaction of patient factors and medication toxicities, appropriate clinical management should include a personalized discussion with each patient to determine the individual treatment plan. Future trials are needed to test novel drugs and establish less toxic approaches to therapy.

Keywords: sarcoidosis, therapeutics, treatment, immunosuppression, granulomatous inflammation

1. Introduction

Sarcoidosis afflicts the lung and thoracic lymph nodes in over 90% of cases [1]. Progressive granulomatous inflammation can lead to diminished pulmonary function, lung fibrosis, and symptoms such as cough and dyspnea. Respiratory failure is the main cause of death or lung transplantation in pulmonary sarcoidosis. Treatment of granulomatous inflammation is targeted at preventing lung dysfunction, improving quality of life, and decreasing mortality. This chapter will review the current basis for therapies that impair development and propagation of granulomatous inflammation in the lung. We review current anti-inflammatory management strategies, as well as evolving research in the field which may lead to new therapeutic strategies. We will also address the difficulties in clinical trials for sarcoidosis and new methods to facilitate development of efficacious therapeutics.

2. Indications for treatment

Granulomas in sarcoidosis are tightly formed clusters of macrophages and monocytes surrounded by CD4+ T-cells and, in lesser presence, B-cells (**Figure 1**). Although the pathophysiology of sarcoidosis is not well-elucidated, current data

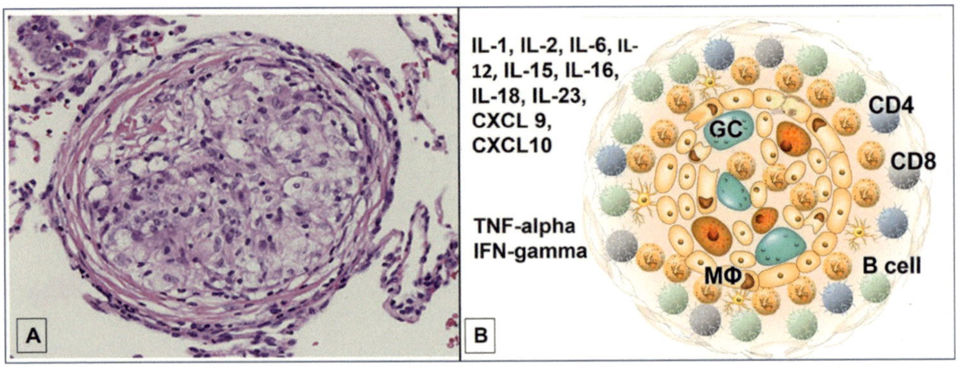

Figure 1.
Sarcoidosis granuloma and associated cytokines and chemokines. A is a histopathologic specimen of a non-necrotizing granuloma from transbronchial lung biopsy and B is a schematic of immune cells and activated cytokines reflecting the predominantly Th-1 immune response. Abbreviations: GC: multi-nucleated giant cell, MΦ: macrophage, TNF: tumor necrosis factor, IFN: interferon, IL: interleukin.

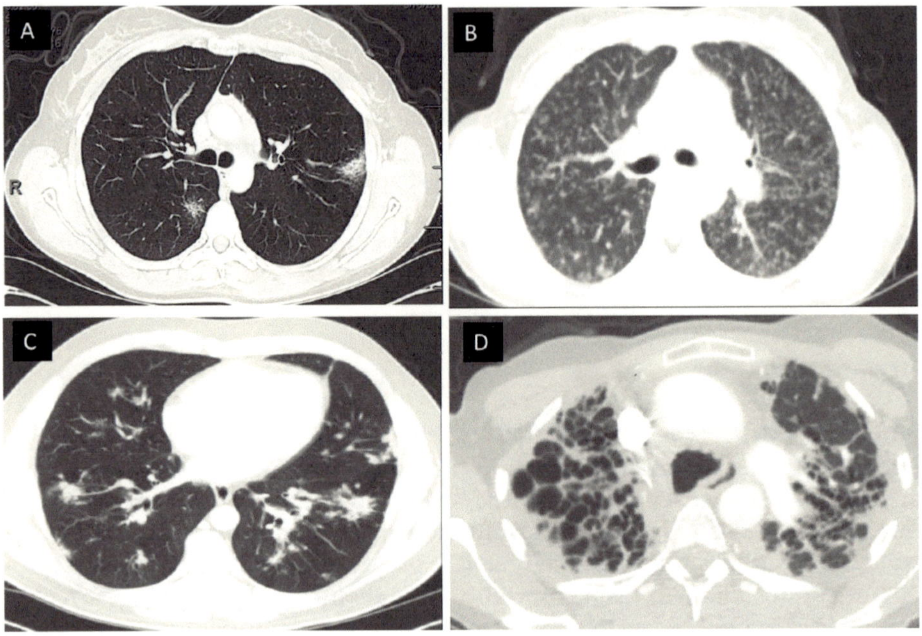

Figure 2.
Pulmonary sarcoidosis. A, B, and C reflect patients with inflammatory granulomatous infiltrates, nodules, and consolidations, whereas D reflects a patient with predominantly fibrotic sarcoidosis of the upper lobes.

suggests a predominant Th-1 immune response with abundant cytokine formation, including tumor necrosis factor (TNF)-alpha and interferon (IFN)-gamma. The driving force is not known, but evidence suggests an environmental antigen in the setting of a genetically predisposed individual. Since eradication of the unknown antigen is not yet possible, current management focuses on interruption of the uncontrolled granulomatous cascade of inflammatory cells which is thought to lead to fibrosis over time.

Not every patient with sarcoidosis necessitates treatment; over half of cases will have spontaneous remission without therapy. Many symptoms, such as fatigue, chronic pain, and cognitive dysfunction, do not respond to immunosuppression and may be confounded by side effects. Additionally, fibrotic sarcoidosis of the lung may not respond to anti-granulomatous therapies (**Figure 2**). Therefore, careful selection of patients is warranted to avoid unnecessary medication use with potentially toxic side effects. Only patients with evidence of significant lung injury, progressive lung function decline, or symptom burden that alters quality life should be considered for therapy. These symptoms of pulmonary sarcoidosis often include cough, chest pain, and/or dyspnea. Given the fairly long span of time over which disability is noted in pulmonary sarcoidosis [2], a period of observation is often employed to determine clinical trajectory if there is no clear indication for immediate therapy (e.g. impending organ damage) and only mild symptoms are present.

3. Treatment options

3.1 Corticosteroids

Large randomized controlled trials guiding therapy are few in the field of sarcoidosis. Corticosteroids remain the mainstay of first-line therapy in the sarcoidosis population. Corticosteroids suppress granulomatous inflammation by broad suppression of inflammatory cytokines such as TNF-alpha and IFN-gamma, prominent factors in the uncontrolled immune response. Proof of long-term mortality benefit and alteration of natural history are lacking, but suppression of the inflammatory response does decrease symptoms and improve imaging and serum biomarkers of disease in many cases of pulmonary sarcoidosis [3, 4].

Corticosteroids tend to be used frequently due to their quick effect and doses can be titrated easily to desired outcomes. However, careful risk/benefit conversations should occur with providers and patients given the potential side effect profile in the long-term management of disease burden. More recent studies have shown that more modest doses of prednisone are equally efficacious as higher doses, particularly for the lung [5]. Generally, dosing of 20–40 mg per day for starting dosage is recommended for pulmonary disease, although an exact dose has not been associated with better outcomes in studies. Therefore, depending on clinical presentation and comorbidities, lower doses can be considered. Doses as low as 15 mg/day have been shown to improve lung infiltrates. Conversely, longer term use of higher doses of prednisone (greater than 40 milligrams (mg) per day) has been shown to increase morbidity and mortality whereas providing little additional physiologic benefit [5]. Additionally, higher corticosteroid use is associated with lower quality of life and increased use of health care resources such as emergency room visits [6]. Corticosteroids can then be tapered to a maintenance dose over a period of weeks to months based on clinical response. In one study, a rapid taper to a low maintenance dose over 3.5 months was effective with less side effects, and most of the pulmonary function benefit was seen within the first month [5]. If corticosteroids cannot be tapered to a dose lower than 10 mg per day, alternative therapies are often considered.

In patients requiring prolonged therapy, in those who have refractory disease, or in those with intolerance or toxicity, corticosteroid-sparing immunomodulators can be considered for additional or alternative therapy. Despite low levels of evidence, recent guidelines support use of these medications in high-risk cases of sarcoidosis [7]. Use of up-front corticosteroid-sparing agents instead of corticosteroids has not been robustly studied, but one retrospective evaluation of methotrexate monotherapy indicated non-inferiority in efficacy as compared to methylprednisolone [8]. Most strategies involving alternative therapies are derived from treatment of other rheumatologic conditions which have historically utilized these medications for suppression of autoimmune-derived inflammation. Safety and use data are often guided by larger trials in other inflammatory diseases (**Table 1**) [9].

3.2 Second-line therapy

Methotrexate (a folic acid antagonist) is the most common second-line therapy recommended in sarcoidosis based on its long-term known safety and efficacy profile in other rheumatologic conditions. Its mechanism in autoimmune disease is likely multifactorial, likely regulating most inflammatory cells either by direct action or indirectly through interruption of various cellular functions. Primarily, the drug involves inhibition of purine and pyrimidine metabolism and suppression of polyamine and amino acid synthesis, thereby suppressing T-cells and B-cells. Other proposed mechanisms via adenosine affect the function of neutrophils and macrophages, altering cytokine function, and preventing immune cell proliferation [10]. Methotrexate has adequate response in approximately 55–80% of patients [11, 12]. The average goal dose of methotrexate is 7.5–15 mg per week, although higher doses can be used if tolerated. The main adverse effects of methotrexate include increased risk of infections, hepatotoxicity, bone marrow suppression, and gastrointestinal side effects; therefore, close monitoring and patient compliance with lab draws are imperative for safe use. Interestingly, in a 'real-world' survey study, patients reported fewer and less bothersome side effects while taking methotrexate as compared to prednisone (49% vs. 78%, respectively) [13].

In cases where methotrexate is not tolerated or ineffective, other corticosteroid-sparing agents are available, with efficacy supported by small trials and case series in sarcoidosis. Leflunomide, another medication used commonly for rheumatoid arthritis, is converted to teriflunomide in the body which then inhibits the mitochondrial enzyme dihydroorotate dehydrogenase. This alteration then inhibits synthesis

First-line
Glucocorticoids
Second-line
Methotrexate
Azathioprine
Mycophenolate
Leflunomide
Third-line
Infliximab
Adalimumab
Other considerations or under study
Rituximab
Repository corticotropin injection
Tofacitinib
Efzofitimod

Table 1.
Stepwise approach to therapy in sarcoidosis.

of ribonucleotide uridine monophosphate pyrimidine (a pyrimidine), and thereby suppressing activated lymphocytes and decreasing proliferation of the T-cells. Dosing ranges from 10 to 20 mg per day. Use of leflunomide is supported by a retrospective look at 76 patients who were prescribed leflunomide after failing alternative immunosuppressives [14]. A significant improvement in forced vital capacity was seen and use allowed tapering of prednisone in these patients. This effect has also been shown in patients who failed methotrexate therapy in another smaller series of patients [15].

Azathioprine is another steroid-sparing agent that is commonly used in sarcoidosis. Its mechanism of action is a purine-mimic antimetabolite that serves to inhibit purine synthesis and diminish the number of circulating B and T lymphocytes, as well as inducing T-cell apoptosis. Dosing ranges from 50 mg per day to 200 mg per day and is often weight-based. Efficacy and side effects are like methotrexate, although azathioprine may have a higher associated rate of infections [16]. In pulmonary sarcoidosis, azathioprine has been shown to improve pulmonary function and to allow tapering of corticosteroids [17]. Similarly, mycophenolate (converted to mycophenolic acid after ingestion) is another drug which inhibits purine nucleotide synthesis in lymphocytes. It is commonly used for treatment of various interstitial lung diseases and can be considered for pulmonary sarcoidosis. Evidence supporting use is based on case series showing a positive steroid-sparing effect with minimal side effects [18–21]. Mycophenolate is given at doses of 1000–3000 mg per day, and an enteric coated variation is available at slightly different dosing range. Antimalarials such as chloroquine or hydroxychloroquine have not been shown to be significantly effective in pulmonary disease but can be used in conjunction with other therapies if concurrent skin involvement or hypercalcemia. This is based upon the drugs' immunomodulatory effect on antigen presentation, T-cell signaling, and interference with inflammatory cytokine production by the lymphocytes [22, 23].

3.3 Third-line therapy

Tumor necrosis factor (TNF) antagonists are recommended as third-line therapy in refractory pulmonary disease [24], with infliximab having the strongest recommendation in recent published guidelines [7]. In a registry cohort of patients with sarcoidosis based out of the United States rheumatology workforce, 12.1% of patients used biologics or targeted disease-modifying antirheumatic drugs [25]. The cytokine, TNF-alpha, plays a large role in the propagation of granulomatous inflammation via macrophage activation. Infliximab (chimeric) and adalimumab (human) are monoclonal antibodies that target TNF itself. Infliximab is given intravenously at a dosing range of 3–5 mg per kilogram at weeks 0, 2, and every 4–8 weeks thereafter. A randomized, placebo-controlled Phase II study of 138 patients showed an improvement of 2.5% in the forced vital capacity compared to placebo, as well as lung radiographic measures and serum biomarkers [26]. This effect was strongest in those with more severe pulmonary disease and those with concurrent extrapulmonary involvement. Controversy on whether this effect was of clinical significance has led to some limitation of its use. However, a more recent retrospective study of 26 patients has shown sustained effects of infliximab on pulmonary infiltrates on long-term follow-up [27]. Interestingly, in another small series of patients who maintained remission after use of third-line infliximab therapy, all had been able to maintain off corticosteroids for at least a year while on infliximab, indicating that perhaps the ability of corticosteroid withdrawal in combination with TNF suppression may be prognostic in the long-term [28]. These results contrast with prior reported high relapse rates after cessation of infliximab, perhaps because of concurrent corticosteroid needs or inadequate duration of therapy [29]. Additionally, because these biologics are only used in refractory cases, it is unclear if delays in effective therapy are associated with worse outcomes [30]. Biosimilars to infliximab also have promising results in small retrospective cohorts to improve lung function, quality of life, and biomarkers [31].

Adalimumab has less robust data in pulmonary disease, but small series have shown it to increase pulmonary function, six-minute walk distance, and radiographic biomarkers in patients with refractory disease [32, 33]. Additionally, it has been shown to have significant efficacy for refractory ocular sarcoidosis, increasing its appeal for multi-system involvement [34, 35]. Adalimumab holds an advantage in that it is a subcutaneous injection (40 mg every 1–2 weeks) that can be self-administered, whereas infliximab requires intravenous infusion. Anti-drug antibodies affecting efficacy can be of concern for all these TNF antagonists [36].

On the other hand, not all biologics have been equally effective. Etanercept, a TNF receptor antagonist was tested in an open label Phase II study for stage 2 and 3 pulmonary sarcoidosis and terminated early due to treatment failure and adverse events [37, 38]. This lack of efficacy in sarcoidosis is further supported by a negative placebo-controlled trial in ocular sarcoidosis [38]. Similarly, ustekinumab and golimumab were ineffective at improving FVC in patients with chronic pulmonary sarcoidosis [39].

3.4 Other potential therapies

Other biologic therapies have shown promise in treatment of granulomatous inflammation in patients with sarcoidosis [40]. Efzofitimod is a novel immunomodulatory fusion protein that selectively binds to neuropilin-2 which is a transmembrane receptor found to be expressed in sarcoid granulomas [41]. In an randomized, double blind, placebo-controlled ascending dose trial of 37 patients with pulmonary sarcoidosis, a greater steroid-sparing effect was seen in the treatment group as compared to the placebo group. Trends towards improvements were seen in quality-of-life measures and lung function that were dose-dependent [42]. The drug was well-tolerated and is being evaluated for further efficacy measures in a larger population.

B-cells in sarcoidosis have also been a plausible target of therapeutics. B-cells have been shown to be involved in granuloma formation, and indirect evidence of heightened B-cell activating factor is present in those with sarcoidosis [43]. Rituximab, a chimeric monoclonal antibody against CD20+ B-cells, was tested in a Phase I/II prospective study of 10 patients with refractory pulmonary sarcoidosis [44]. Five of those patients improved their forced vital capacity (FVC) by at least 5% and five of the patients had an improvement in 6 minute walk distance by 30 meters (seven patients total with either or both outcomes). However, in follow-up, 2 patients had progressive respiratory failure and one was hospitalized for infectious pneumonia, making broad use less clear for rituximab until further studies can be performed.

Tofacitinib, a JAK inhibitor, was found to be efficacious in an open label study of 10 patients with moderate to severe cutaneous lesions. Positron emission tomography (PET) scans in these patients also showed marked decrease (>50%) in avidity of lung lesions in five of eight patients with pulmonary sarcoidosis [45]. Repository corticotropin injection has also undergone testing as an immune modulator in sarcoidosis in a phase IV placebo-controlled trial. Its anti-inflammatory effects are thought to be mediated by the melanocortin receptors present on the immune cells which thereby decrease the production of pro-inflammatory cytokines. Steroid-sparing effect was overall like the placebo group; however, corticosteroids were tapered in a faster manner in the treatment group [46]. Non-significant trends were seen in secondary endpoints, including pulmonary function and quality of life. Smaller case series and retrospective reviews have supported a steroid-sparing effect, albeit with some toxicity [47, 48]. Larger, more robust studies are needed to determine future use of these drugs. Other anti-inflammatory agents under study include anti-GM-CSF antibodies, monoclonal antibodies against IL-18, and nicotine, a modulator of the T-cell regulatory pathways [49]. Nintedanib, an anti-fibrotic agent, has been approved for all types of progressive fibrosis of the lung via the INBUILD trial which included a small number of patients with sarcoidosis. Whether it has any anti-inflammatory properties is unknown for sarcoidosis but is a consideration for progressive fibrotic disease despite immunosuppression [50].

3.5 Inhaled therapy

Inhaled therapies are also used in pulmonary sarcoidosis, although primarily for treatment of cough, exacerbations, or more mild airway inflammation. An early randomized controlled trial showed that high dose inhaled corticosteroids were not effective in treatment of symptoms, X-rays, pulmonary function, or serum biomarkers in stage 1–3 sarcoidosis, albeit only 21 patients were included, and many had regression of disease without therapy at all [51]. Therefore, the role of inhaled therapies in certain sub-phenotypes is still unknown.

4. Considerations for treatment decisions

4.1 Comorbid conditions

The decisions of when to treat, with what medication, and for how long is based both on clinical presentation and a personalized discussion between patient and provider regarding the likelihood of clinical benefit in the setting of comorbidities, medication side effects, as well as patient preferences. The presence of comorbidities can also contribute greatly to the choice of therapy. Corticosteroids can exacerbate diabetes, glaucoma, hypertension, obesity, and fluid retention, whereas increasing risk of osteoporosis, bone fractures, and cataracts. They have also been associated with lower health-related quality of life, even when adjusted for severity of disease [52]. Concurrent medication can also significantly interact with several corticosteroid-sparing medications. Similarly, renal or liver dysfunction may require dose-adjustment of medications. Use of alcohol should also be evaluated and incorporated into therapy decisions, as alcohol can increase risk of hepatotoxicity when taking methotrexate.

4.2 Reproductive health

The possibility or desire of pregnancy should also be considered in choosing an immunosuppressive agent [53]. Methotrexate and mycophenolate are associated with increased risk of pregnancy loss and teratogenicity. Due to teratogenicity of leflunomide in mice studies, it is also not recommended in pregnancy. Mycophenolate, methotrexate, and leflunomide are contraindicated in women who are breast-feeding. Azathioprine, corticosteroids, and TNF-antagonists have more favorable profiles in terms of teratogenicity; however, risks and benefits should be discussed when prescribing this in pregnancy. Side effects such as hyperglycemia, hypertension, and increased infection risk can be heightened in pregnancy.

4.3 Pharmacogenomics

Some of the heterogenous efficacy of corticosteroid-sparing drugs such as methotrexate and leflunomide can be explained by genetic determinants of medication response [54–56]. Similarly, genetic polymorphisms of the genes responsible for metabolism of azathioprine (thiopurine S-methyltransferase and nucleoside triphosphate diphosphatase) have been associated with medication-related toxicity, including bone marrow suppression and hepatotoxicity [56]. However, testing for these polymorphisms is not universally agreed upon, just under half of patients with toxicity have no known genetic predisposition. Hence, close monitoring of liver function and blood counts are required in all patients who are prescribed azathioprine. Based on these potential pharmacogenomic traits, consideration of switching steroid-sparing medications is warranted if one has toxicity or lacks efficacy.

4.4 Treatment non-response

In addition to genetic variation in medication response, cases of 'refractory' disease could indicate other potential reasons for failure. If a patient is not responding, alternative diagnoses should be entertained. Additionally, non-adherence to medication can also play a role, and can occur due to financial constraints, high side effect profiles of medications, inaccessibility to health care resources (e.g. lab draws), or burdensome limitations to a patient's work or eating schedules.

5. Duration of treatment and follow-up

Duration of treatment to maintain remission varies, but approximately 1 year is a reasonable approach and can depend greatly on severity of disease, extrapulmonary involvement, and medication tolerance. Shorter courses have been associated with increased rates of relapse, both with corticosteroids and infliximab [57]. Similarly, use of corticosteroids has been associated with increased relapse rate, bringing up the concept that the granuloma may be an adaptive response [58]. Longer courses have been associated with better outcomes in lung function, radiographs, and symptoms. There are no validated predictors of relapse, and it is unclear on how steroid-sparing agents affect relapse rate.

Ongoing efforts between a patient and provider to decrease therapy at regular intervals to lowest effective doses are warranted. Improvements of pulmonary function and symptoms after treatment appear to happen most prominently in the first month, with additional smaller effects seen over a period of 3 months, arguing that tapering of corticosteroids early and finding the lowest maintenance doses of medications thereafter may help alleviate long-term medication toxicity [5].

6. Future directions in therapeutics

Clinical trials in sarcoidosis are difficult to perform due to rarity of the disease, uncertain clinical course (many improve spontaneously), heterogeneity of disease presentation, and inadequate outcome measures of disease response. Furthermore, despite known long-term toxicities associated with corticosteroids, it is difficult to test novel therapeutics in direct comparison in placebo-controlled trials. For this reason, outcomes such as steroid-sparing effects or radiographic biomarkers have become more common. Standardization of outcomes across trials and development of personalized biomarkers to predict disease activity would greatly aid appropriate inclusion criteria to increase efficiency of clinical studies and more precisely identify clinical improvements [59]. Current work in transcriptomics and radiomics hold promise for these outcome measures [60]. Despite these difficulties, future trials are imperative to develop therapies that can alleviate the severe burden of disease and medication side effects, avoid lung transplantation, and decrease mortality.

7. Conclusions

Sarcoidosis is a complex disease with heterogeneous clinical course and limited clinical trials by which to guide therapy. Treatment should only be considered in those with significant symptoms, to prevent or alleviate organ damage, and to protect from sarcoidosis-associated mortality. Glucocorticoids continue to be first-line therapy, but corticosteroid-sparing medications should be considered for patients requiring prolonged therapy, those who have side effects or toxicity related to steroids, or for those in whom corticosteroids cannot be tapered to a reasonable dose. Despite low levels of evidence for most corticosteroid-sparing immune modulators, these options can be considered. Future trials are needed to test novel drugs and establish less toxic approaches to therapy. Last, appropriate clinical management should include a personalized discussion with each patient to determine each individual treatment plan.

Conflict of interest

The author declares no conflict of interest.

Author details

Alicia K. Gerke
Department of Internal Medicine, Division of Pulmonary and Critical Care,
University of Iowa, Iowa City, Iowa, USA

*Address all correspondence to: alicia-gerke@uiowa.edu

References

[1] Baughman RP, Teirstein AS, Judson MA, Rossman MD, Yeager H Jr, Bresnitz EA, et al. Clinical characteristics of patients in a case control study of sarcoidosis. American Journal of Respiratory and Critical Care Medicine. 2001;**164**(10 Pt 1):1885-1889

[2] Takada K, Ina Y, Noda M, Sato T, Yamamoto M, Morishita M. The clinical course and prognosis of patients with severe, moderate or mild sarcoidosis. Journal of Clinical Epidemiology. 1993;**46**(4):359-366

[3] Pietinalho A, Tukiainen P, Haahtela T, Persson T, Selroos O, Finnish Pulmonary Sarcoidosis Study G. Early treatment of stage II sarcoidosis improves 5-year pulmonary function. Chest. 2002;**121**(1):24-31

[4] Gibson GJ, Prescott RJ, Muers MF, Middleton WG, Mitchell DN, Connolly CK, et al. British Thoracic Society Sarcoidosis study: Effects of long term corticosteroid treatment. Thorax. 1996;**51**(3):238-247

[5] Broos CE, Poell LHC, Looman CWN, In 't Veen J, Grootenboers M, Heller R, et al. No evidence found for an association between prednisone dose and FVC change in newly-treated pulmonary sarcoidosis. Respiratory Medicine. 2018;**138S**:S31-SS7

[6] Judson MA, Chaudhry H, Louis A, Lee K, Yucel R. The effect of corticosteroids on quality of life in a sarcoidosis clinic: The results of a propensity analysis. Respiratory Medicine. 2015;**109**(4):526-531

[7] Baughman RP, Valeyre D, Korsten P, Mathioudakis AG, Wuyts WA, Wells A, et al. ERS clinical practice guidelines on treatment of sarcoidosis. The European Respiratory Journal. 2021;**58**(6):2004079

[8] Gavrysyuk V, Merenkova I, Dziublyk Y, Morska N, Pendalchuk N, Bychenko O, et al. Efficacy and tolerability of methotrexate and methylprednisolone in a comparative assessment of the primary and long-term outcomes in patients with pulmonary sarcoidosis. Diagnostics (Basel). 2021;**11**(7):1289

[9] Moreland LW, O'Dell JR, Paulus HE, Curtis JR, Bathon JM, St Clair EW, et al. A randomized comparative effectiveness study of oral triple therapy versus etanercept plus methotrexate in early aggressive rheumatoid arthritis: The treatment of Early Aggressive Rheumatoid Arthritis Trial. Arthritis and Rheumatism. 2012;**64**(9):2824-2835

[10] Cronstein BN, Aune TM. Methotrexate and its mechanisms of action in inflammatory arthritis. Nature Reviews Rheumatology. 2020;**16**(3):145-154

[11] Fang C, Zhang Q, Wang N, Jing X, Xu Z. Effectiveness and tolerability of methotrexate in pulmonary sarcoidosis: A single center real-world study. Sarcoidosis, Vasculitis, and Diffuse Lung Diseases. 2019;**36**(3):217-227

[12] Goljan-Geremek A, Bednarek M, Franczuk M, Puscinska E, Nowinski A, Czystowska M, et al. Methotrexate as a single agent for treating pulmonary sarcoidosis: A single centre real-life prospective study. Pneumonologia i Alergologia Polska. 2014;**82**(6):518-533

[13] Kahlmann V, Moor CC, Veltkamp M, Wijsenbeek MS. Patient reported side-effects of prednisone and methotrexate

in a real-world sarcoidosis population. Chronic Respiratory Disease. 2021;**18**:14799731211031935

[14] Sahoo DH, Bandyopadhyay D, Xu M, Pearson K, Parambil JG, Lazar CA, et al. Effectiveness and safety of leflunomide for pulmonary and extrapulmonary sarcoidosis. The European Respiratory Journal. 2011;**38**(5):1145-1150

[15] Baughman RP, Lower EE. Leflunomide for chronic sarcoidosis. Sarcoidosis, Vasculitis, and Diffuse Lung Diseases. 2004;**21**(1):43-48

[16] Pasipanodya JG. Comparative effectiveness of methotrexate versus methylprednisolone in treatment naive pulmonary sarcoidosis patients. Diagnostics (Basel). 2021;**11**(8):1401

[17] Vorselaars ADM, Wuyts WA, Vorselaars VMM, Zanen P, Deneer VHM, Veltkamp M, et al. Methotrexate vs azathioprine in second-line therapy of sarcoidosis. Chest. 2013;**144**(3):805-812

[18] Hamzeh N, Voelker A, Forssen A, Gottschall EB, Rose C, Mroz P, et al. Efficacy of mycophenolate mofetil in sarcoidosis. Respiratory Medicine. 2014;**108**(11):1663-1669

[19] Brill AK, Ott SR, Geiser T. Effect and safety of mycophenolate mofetil in chronic pulmonary sarcoidosis: A retrospective study. Respiration. 2013;**86**(5):376-383

[20] Vonk MC, Smith V, Sfikakis PP, Cutolo M, Del Galdo F, Seibold JR. Pharmacological treatments for SSc-ILD: Systematic review and critical appraisal of the evidence. Autoimmunity Reviews. 2021;**20**(12):102978

[21] van den Bosch L, Luppi F, Ferrara G, Mura M. Immunomodulatory treatment of interstitial lung disease. Therapeutic Advances in Respiratory Disease. 2022;**16**:17534666221117002

[22] Schrezenmeier E, Dorner T. Mechanisms of action of hydroxychloroquine and chloroquine: Implications for rheumatology. Nature Reviews Rheumatology. 2020;**16**(3):155-166

[23] Sharma OP. Effectiveness of chloroquine and hydroxychloroquine in treating selected patients with sarcoidosis with neurological involvement. Archives of Neurology. 1998;**55**(9):1248-1254

[24] Rahaghi FF, Baughman RP, Saketkoo LA, Sweiss NJ, Barney JB, Birring SS, et al. Delphi consensus recommendations for a treatment algorithm in pulmonary sarcoidosis. European Respiratory Review. 2020;**29**(155):190146

[25] Hammam N, Evans M, Morgan E, Reimold A, Anastasiou C, Kay JL, et al. Treatment of sarcoidosis in US rheumatology practices: Data from the American College of Rheumatology's Rheumatology Informatics System for Effectiveness (RISE) Registry. Arthritis Care & Research (Hoboken). 2022;**74**(3):371-376

[26] Baughman RP, Drent M, Kavuru M, Judson MA, Costabel U, du Bois R, et al. Infliximab therapy in patients with chronic sarcoidosis and pulmonary involvement. American Journal of Respiratory and Critical Care Medicine. 2006;**174**(7):795-802

[27] Russell E, Luk F, Manocha S, Ho T, O'Connor C, Hussain H. Long term follow-up of infliximab efficacy in pulmonary and extra-pulmonary sarcoidosis refractory to conventional therapy. Seminars in Arthritis and Rheumatism. 2013;**43**(1):119-124

[28] Yee AMF. Durable medication-free remission of sarcoidosis following discontinuation of anti-tumor necrosis factor-alpha therapy. Respiratory Medicine. 2023;**206**:107055

[29] Baughman RP, Judson MA. Relapses of sarcoidosis: What are they and can we predict who will get them? The European Respiratory Journal. 2014;**43**(2):337-339

[30] Vorselaars ADM, Culver DA. Hit-hard and early versus step-up treatment in severe sarcoidosis. Current Opinion in Pulmonary Medicine. 2022;**28**(5):461-467

[31] Schimmelpennink MC, Vorselaars ADM, van Beek FT, CrommelinHA,DeneerVHM,KeijsersRGM, et al. Efficacy and safety of infliximab biosimilar Inflectra((R)) in severe sarcoidosis. Respiratory Medicine. 2018;**138S**:S7-S13

[32] Kamphuis LS, Lam-Tse WK, Dik WA, van Daele PL, van Biezen P, Kwekkeboom DJ, et al. Efficacy of adalimumab in chronically active and symptomatic patients with sarcoidosis. American Journal of Respiratory and Critical Care Medicine. 2011;**184**(10):1214-1216

[33] Sweiss NJ, Noth I, Mirsaeidi M, Zhang W, Naureckas ET, Hogarth DK, et al. Efficacy results of a 52-week trial of adalimumab in the treatment of refractory sarcoidosis. Sarcoidosis, Vasculitis, and Diffuse Lung Diseases. 2014;**31**(1):46-54

[34] Erckens RJ, Mostard RL, Wijnen PA, Schouten JS, Drent M. Adalimumab successful in sarcoidosis patients with refractory chronic non-infectious uveitis. Graefe's Archive for Clinical and Experimental Ophthalmology. 2012;**250**(5):713-720

[35] Riancho-Zarrabeitia L, Calvo-Rio V, Blanco R, Mesquida M, Adan AM, Herreras JM, et al. Anti-TNF-alpha therapy in refractory uveitis associated with sarcoidosis: Multicenter study of 17 patients. Seminars in Arthritis and Rheumatism. 2015;**45**(3):361-368

[36] Radstake TR, Svenson M, Eijsbouts AM, van den Hoogen FH, Enevold C, van Riel PL, et al. Formation of antibodies against infliximab and adalimumab strongly correlates with functional drug levels and clinical responses in rheumatoid arthritis. Annals of the Rheumatic Diseases. 2009;**68**(11):1739-1745

[37] Utz JP, Limper AH, Kalra S, Specks U, Scott JP, Vuk-Pavlovic Z, et al. Etanercept for the treatment of stage II and III progressive pulmonary sarcoidosis. Chest. 2003;**124**(1):177-185

[38] Baughman RP, Lower EE, Bradley DA, Raymond LA, Kaufman A. Etanercept for refractory ocular sarcoidosis: Results of a double-blind randomized trial. Chest. 2005;**128**(2):1062-1047

[39] Judson MA, Baughman RP, Costabel U, Drent M, Gibson KF, Raghu G, et al. Safety and efficacy of ustekinumab or golimumab in patients with chronic sarcoidosis. The European Respiratory Journal. 2014;**44**(5):1296-1307

[40] Plichta J, Kuna P, Panek M. Biologic drugs in the treatment of chronic inflammatory pulmonary diseases: Recent developments and future perspectives. Frontiers in Immunology. 2023;**14**:1207641

[41] Baughman RP, Niranjan V, Walker G, Burkart C, Paz S, Chong Y, et al. Efzofitimod: A novel anti-inflammatory agent for sarcoidosis.

Sarcoidosis, Vasculitis, and Diffuse Lung Diseases. 2023;**40**(1):e2023011

[42] Culver DA, Aryal S, Barney J, Hsia CCW, James WE, Maier LA, et al. Efzofitimod for the treatment of pulmonary sarcoidosis. Chest. 2023;**163**(4):881-890

[43] Kamphuis LS, van Zelm MC, Lam KH, Rimmelzwaan GF, Baarsma GS, Dik WA, et al. Perigranuloma localization and abnormal maturation of B cells: Emerging key players in sarcoidosis? American Journal of Respiratory and Critical Care Medicine. 2013;**187**(4):406-416

[44] Sweiss NJ, Lower EE, Mirsaeidi M, Dudek S, Garcia JG, Perkins D, et al. Rituximab in the treatment of refractory pulmonary sarcoidosis. The European Respiratory Journal. 2014;**43**(5):1525-1528

[45] Damsky W, Young BD, Sloan B, Miller EJ, Obando JA, King B. Treatment of multiorgan sarcoidosis with tofacitinib. ACR Open Rheumatology. 2020;**2**(2):106-109

[46] Mirsaeidi M, Baughman RP. Repository corticotropin injection for the treatment of pulmonary sarcoidosis: A narrative review. Pulmonary Therapy. 2022;**8**(1):43-55

[47] Baughman RP, Sweiss N, Keijsers R, Birring SS, Shipley R, Saketkoo LA, et al. Repository corticotropin for chronic pulmonary sarcoidosis. Lung. 2017;**195**(3):313-322

[48] Chopra I, Qin Y, Kranyak J, Gallagher JR, Heap K, Carroll S, et al. Repository corticotropin injection in patients with advanced symptomatic sarcoidosis: Retrospective analysis of medical records. Therapeutic Advances in Respiratory Disease. 2019;**13**:1753466619888127

[49] Obi ON, Saketkoo LA, Russell AM, Baughman RP. Sarcoidosis: Updates on therapeutic drug trials and novel treatment approaches. Frontiers in Medicine. 2022;**9**:991783

[50] Wells AU, Flaherty KR, Brown KK, Inoue Y, Devaraj A, Richeldi L, et al. Nintedanib in patients with progressive fibrosing interstitial lung diseases-subgroup analyses by interstitial lung disease diagnosis in the INBUILD trial: A randomised, double-blind, placebo-controlled, parallel-group trial. The Lancet Respiratory Medicine. 2020;**8**(5):453-460

[51] Milman N, Graudal N, Grode G, Munch E. No effect of high-dose inhaled steroids in pulmonary sarcoidosis: A double-blind, placebo-controlled study. Journal of Internal Medicine. 1994;**236**(3):285-290

[52] Cox CE, Donohue JF, Brown CD, Kataria YP, Judson MA. Health-related quality of life of persons with sarcoidosis. Chest. 2004;**125**(3):997-1004

[53] Sammaritano LR, Bermas BL, Chakravarty EE, Chambers C, Clowse MEB, Lockshin MD, et al. 2020 American College of Rheumatology Guideline for the Management of Reproductive Health in Rheumatic and Musculoskeletal Diseases. Arthritis & Rhematology. 2020;**72**(4):529-556

[54] Qiu Q, Huang J, Shu X, Fan H, Zhou Y, Xiao C. Polymorphisms and pharmacogenomics for the clinical efficacy of methotrexate in patients with rheumatoid arthritis: A systematic review and meta-analysis. Scientific Reports. 2017;7:44015

[55] Bohanec Grabar P, Rozman B, Tomsic M, Suput D, Logar D, Dolzan V.

Genetic polymorphism of CYP1A2 and the toxicity of leflunomide treatment in rheumatoid arthritis patients. European Journal of Clinical Pharmacology. 2008;**64**(9):871-876

[56] Lennard L, Van Loon JA, Weinshilboum RM. Pharmacogenetics of acute azathioprine toxicity: Relationship to thiopurine methyltransferase genetic polymorphism. Clinical Pharmacology and Therapeutics. 1989;**46**(2):149-154

[57] Vorselaars AD, Verwoerd A, van Moorsel CH, Keijsers RG, Rijkers GT, Grutters JC. Prediction of relapse after discontinuation of infliximab therapy in severe sarcoidosis. The European Respiratory Journal. 2014;**43**(2):602-609

[58] Judson MA, Adelstein E, Fish KM, Feustel PJ, Yucel R, Preston S, et al. Outcomes of prednisone-tapering regimens for cardiac sarcoidosis: A retrospective analysis demonstrating a benefit of infliximab. Respiratory Medicine. 2022;**203**:107004

[59] Hena KM, Patterson KC. Making progress in clinical trials in sarcoidosis. Chest. 2023;**164**(3):682-685

[60] Francesqui J, Marrades P, Sellares J. Personalized medicine in sarcoidosis: Unravelling biomarkers for targeted care. Current Opinion in Pulmonary Medicine. 2023;**29**(5):478-484